Visual Reference Guides

Herbal Remedies

ANDREW CHEVALLIER

US CONSULTANT

DAVID KEIFER

METRO BOOKS
NEW YORK

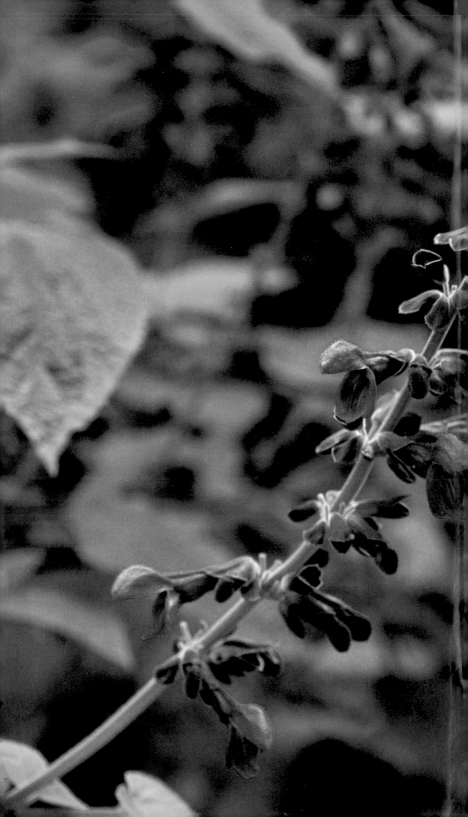

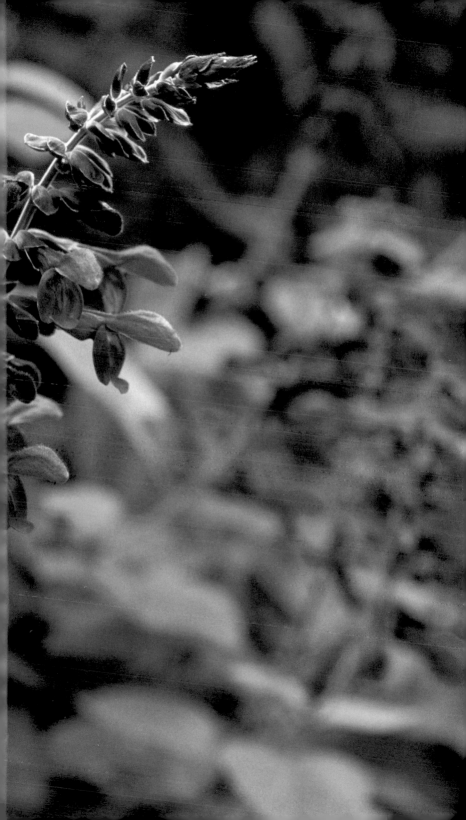

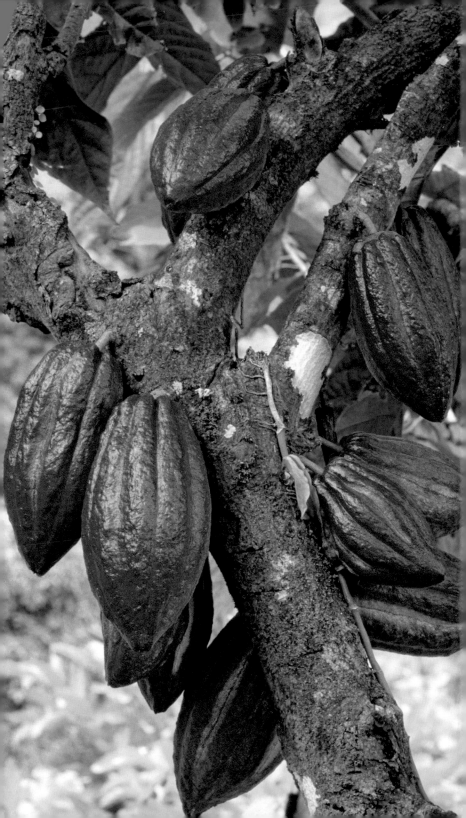

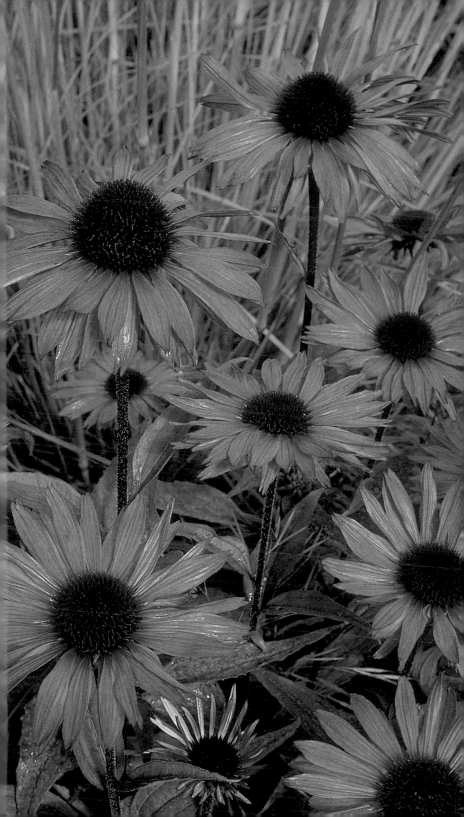

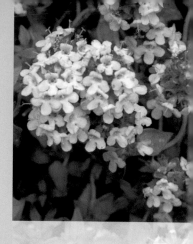

Designers	Arunesh Talapatra
	Tannishtha Chakraborty
Editors	Dipali Singh, Aditi Ray,
	Pankhoori Sinha
Senior Editor	Jennifer Latham
US Editor	Christy Lusiak
Senior Art Editor	Anne Fisher
Managing Art Editor	Marianne Markham
Managing Editor	Penny Warren
Picture Research	Myriam Megharbi,
	Romaine Werblow, Claire
	Bowers, Lucy Claxton
DTP Designers	Sunil Sharma,
	Harish Aggarwal, Govind
	Mittal, Pushpak Tyagi
Production Controller	Rebecca Short

Metro Books
122 Fifth Avenue
New York, NY 10011

ISBN 978-1-4351-2131-7

Cataloging in-Publication data is available from the
Library of Congress

Colour reproduction by Media Development and Printing, UK
Printed and bound in China by LRex

1   3   5   7   9   10   8   6   4   2

Important notice Do not try to self-diagnose or attempt
self-treatment for serious long-term problems without first
consulting a qualified herbal medicine expert or doctor. Do not
take any herb without first checking the cautions in the relevant
herb entry and the guidelines in Safety and Quality pp.40–51.
Do not exceed recommended dosages. Always consult a
professional if symptoms persist. If taking prescribed medicines,
seek professional advice before using herbal remedies.

Foreword 8
Introduction 10

Chapter One

WHAT IS HERBAL MEDICINE?

Why use herbal
remedies? *14*

Herbal health *16*

Are herbal remedies
safe? *18*

How remedies work *20*

Around the world *22*

Chapter Two

USING HERBAL REMEDIES

Making herbal
medicines *26*

Types of
herbal remedy *30*

Herbal remedies at
home *34*

The home herbal *36*

The herb
garden *38*

CONTENTS

Chapter Three
SAFETY AND QUALITY

Safety concerns 42

Dosage and sensible use 44

Pregnancy and after 46

Tips for home use 48

How to buy remedies 50

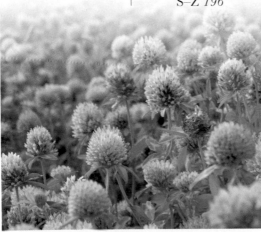

Chapter Four
A–Z OF HERBAL REMEDIES

A–F 54

G–L 135

M–R 162

S–Z 196

Chapter Five
COMMON HEALTH PROBLEMS

Head 259

Throat, chest, and lungs 261

Digestion 262

Circulation and heart 263

Blood, metabolic 264

Bladder and urinary tract 265

Joints, muscles, and bone 266

Skin 267

Women's health problems 268

Men's health problems 270

Mental and emotional problems 271

Promoting health and performance 272

Supporting immune function 272

Children's common health problems 273

Glossary 276

Resources 278

Index 280

Acknowledgments 288

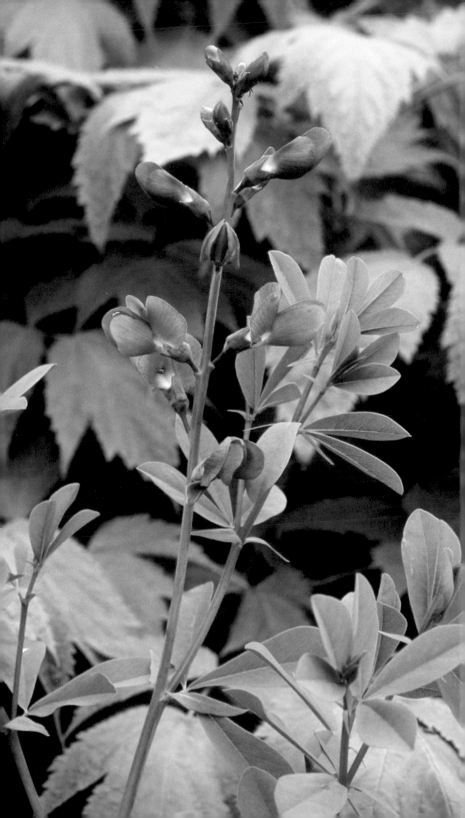

FOREWORD

The last decade has seen a rapid increase in the publication of books on herbal medicine. However, it is rare to find one, such as this, that incorporates details of over-the-counter remedies, written for the general public by a practicing herbal practitioner. Andrew Chevallier brings to this book years of experience in clinical practice and book authorship (he is the author of the *Encyclopaedia of Medicinal Plants*—also published by Dorling Kindersley). Andrew is a well-known and respected member of the herbal fraternity in the UK, having been in the past President of the National Institute of Medical Herbalists.

The origins of the use of herbs dates back to prehistoric times, and their traditional medicinal use continues in all cultural groups throughout the world. Many modern medicines were inspired by constituents found in traditional medicinal plants, and some modern drugs are still isolated from plant materials. However, the big difference between herbal and modern medicine is that while modern medicines comprise single chemicals, nature has endowed each herb with a spectrum of active components, which work synergistically to produce a healing effect that cannot be replicated from single components.

Over the last twenty years there has been a resurgence of interest in the use of herbal medicine. There are several reasons for this, but the main ones are an increasing realization of the limits of modern medicine, particularly in the treatment of chronic disease; fear of adverse side effects of prescription drugs, and the increasing support for the medicinal use of plants from modern clinical research. However, herbal medicine need not be an alternative to modern medicine. Indeed, most herbs are mild medicines that work well alongside prescription drugs. Despite media "hype," true herb–drug interactions are few and these are clearly indicated, as appropriate, in this book.

Although the treatment of chronic disease always requires professional advice, with minor health complaints there is a lot you can do for yourself using over-the-counter herbal preparations. The key to finding successful natural remedies is knowing what you are doing and why. This book provides the necessary guidance. Eating a healthy diet is fundamental to maintaining good health, but herbs have a special role to play when minor health problems arise.

ELDERFLOWER

DR ANN WALKER
PHD MNIMH MCPP RNUTR
Senior Lecturer in Human Nutrition,
University of Reading
Director, The Herb Society (UK)
October 2006

MEDICINAL LORE
Knowledge of medicinal plants often comes down to us from longstanding traditional use. Wild indigo root (*Baptista tinctoria*) was used by Native Americans to bathe cuts and treat rattlesnake bites.

IN RECENT YEARS, PEOPLE HAVE REDISCOVERED THE NUMEROUS BENEFITS THAT HERBAL MEDICINE HAS TO OFFER. HERBS SUCH AS ECHINACEA, GARLIC, AND GINGER HAVE BECOME FAMILIAR AND WELL-USED HOUSEHOLD REMEDIES, WHILE THE RANGE OF HERBS AND HERBAL PRODUCTS AVAILABLE OVER-THE-COUNTER HAS GROWN TREMENDOUSLY.

Several hundred remedies, from arnica (*Arnica montana*) to withania (*Withania somnifera*), are now readily found in health food stores and pharmacies, while thousands are available on the Internet. The opportunities to find safe and effective herbal remedies for home treatment may never have been better. And whether they are taken to relieve common health problems, to prevent illness, or to enhance performance, herbal remedies—when used wisely—will work to improve health and vitality.

While choice provides opportunity, it often comes with a sting in its tail! Walking down the aisles of a health food store, past row upon row of competing products, can be a bewildering experience. If you want a remedy for sinus congestion or period pains, how do you make your choice and decide what to buy? If you know that you want elderflower (*Sambucus nigra*) for sinus congestion, or white peony (*Paeonia lactiflora*) for period pains, many questions still arise. How do you know it will work? What type of preparation is best—tablet, tea, or tincture? Are there safety issues? What is good value for money?

Would a single herb product or a combination be most appropriate? Will it conflict with other medication you are taking?

Answering these questions in detail is beyond the scope of any one book, but *Herbal Remedies* aims to provide you with the essential information to answer such questions, to choose safe and appropriate herbal remedies, and to put them to good use.

Unlike synthetic medicines, herbal remedies are harvested from fields and forests all over the world. Their healing, therapeutic activity is simply one aspect of the plant world's bountiful and generous relationship with animal life on our planet. With its many photographs and illustrations, this book reveals just a little of the beauty and variety to be found in medicinal plants, and encourages a greater awareness of the need to protect and conserve them in the wild. It is written in the hope that it will open up the world of herbal medicine for you and enable you to use herbal remedies to good effect.

HERBAL STORES
Herbal remedies are available all over the world and in many different forms. It pays to buy from stores that specialize in herbal medicine, with well-trained staff who can give sound advice.

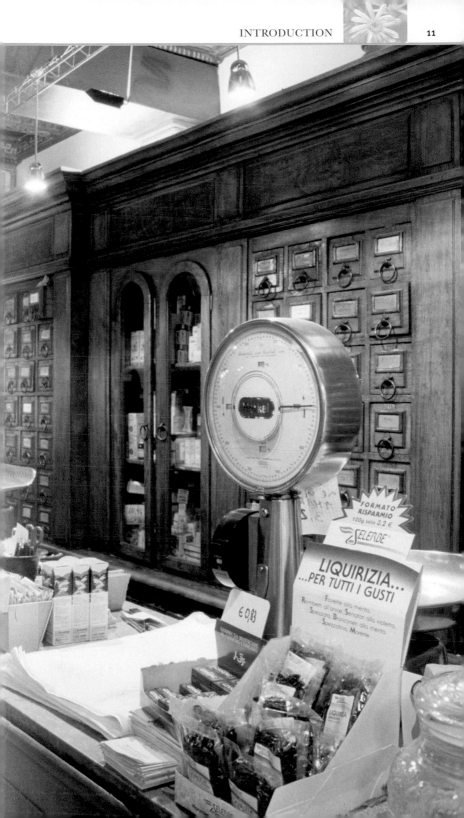

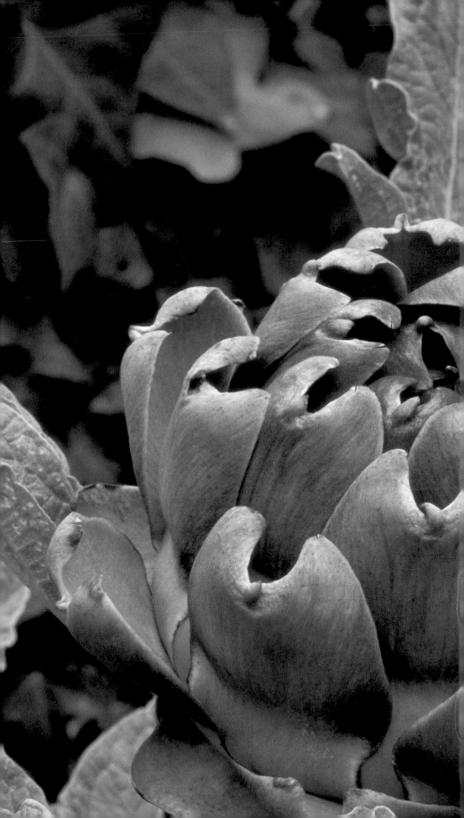

WHAT IS HERBAL MEDICINE?

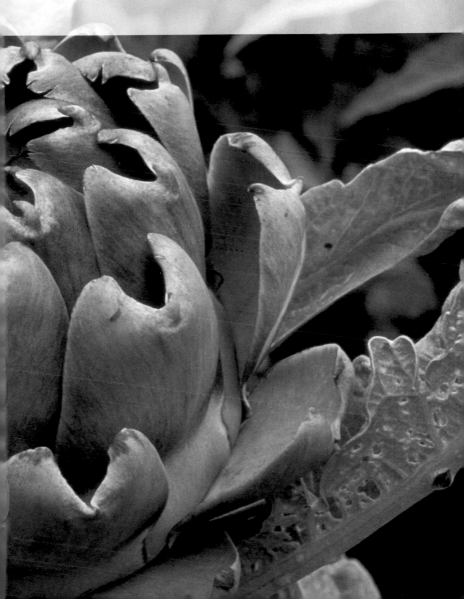

WHY USE HERBAL REMEDIES?

When confronted by ill health, human beings have always sought medicines from the natural world, in particular from plants. Today, we have the opportunity to combine traditional knowledge of herbal medicine with the clarity that scientific research can provide.

Back to nature

Strange as it may seem to us today, one reason why herbal medicines fell out of favor among doctors and scientists in the 19th and 20th centuries was because they were natural! While conventional medicines, such as aspirin, are mostly made up of single chemical compounds, herbal medicines may contain many hundreds of different constituents. As a consequence, it can be a daunting task for researchers to discover how an herb works and to identify the constituents responsible. No wonder it has been found much more straightforward to focus attention on single chemicals, which, if necessary, can be extracted and purified from medicinal plants.

Herbal medicines are also viewed with suspicion because they are prone to natural variation. Different seasons produce slightly different crops. As one authority has put it, good quality in herbal medicine is not too different from good quality in wine. As in the case of grapevines, medicinal plants need to be tended with care, harvested at the right time, and processed appropriately to achieve the best results. Even then, some crops will be better than others.

The most serious complaint laid against herbal medicines, however, is that they can easily be adulterated. To most people, one pile of dried green leaves looks very much like another. If one is worth five times more than the other, the temptation will always be there to "cut" the more valuable one, or to substitute a cheaper variety. In order to prevent poor-quality material from being sold and to guarantee safety, quality control is essential.

WHY USE HERBS?

If herbal medicines are so complicated and variable, why use them? Some of the strengths of herbal medicines are listed below, and you will find examples of them throughout this book.

- Human beings have evolved alongside plants, using them as food and medicine.
- Herbal remedies are often dilute and can be adjusted to individual strength.
- They usually work with the body's own physiological processes.
- When used sensibly, they have an enviable safety record.
- Medical research endorses a number of key herbal remedies where safety and effectiveness have been established.
- Other remedies have longstanding traditional use as evidence of their efficacy.
- They can be safely self-administered in minor acute and chronic conditions.
- Some remedies can be taken long-term in low doses.
- Many remedies can be taken to prevent illness or enhance performance.
- As natural products, they are a permanently renewable resource. When grown organically, they can have a positive impact on the environment.

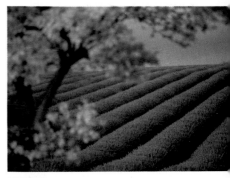

LAVENDER
Herbal medicines such as lavender (*Lavandula officinalis*) are natural products and vary in quality in the same way as is found in wine.

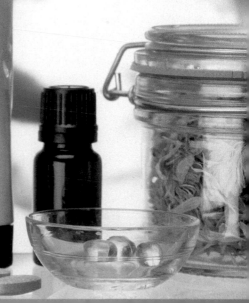

THE HERBAL MEDICINE CHEST
Medicinal plants can be processed in many different ways. The most common examples are teas, tinctures, and extracts made into capsules and tablets.

HERBAL HEALTH

This section looks at the broad picture of the way in which herbal remedies may be employed. For detailed advice on the self-treatment of particular problems, please refer to the Common Health Problems section on pp.256–275.

Herbal remedies can be safely used to:
• Treat common acute problems, for example coughs, headaches, and skin rashes.
• Treat chronic problems, for example mild depression, arthritis, and varicose veins.
• Prevent illness.
• Enhance health.
Although they are natural, herbal remedies are medicines and can therefore cause side effects. For best results, they need to be used sensibly and with respect. They also need to be used with an awareness of what they cannot do!

MINOR ACUTE PROBLEMS

Herbal remedies are well suited to treating everyday health problems, though the standard caution about self, or home, treatment always applies: if you are in doubt, seek immediate professional advice, especially where unwell children are concerned. Relief for conditions such as headache, sore throat, cough, gas, and bloating can occur quickly, although gradual, ongoing improvement in symptoms is more common with herbal medicine. Warm teas

and diluted tinctures can be particularly helpful. For simple problems, treatment for a few days will be sufficient. Skin problems such as minor burns, grazes, and rashes can be treated topically.

Example Symptoms of sore throat and hoarseness suggesting the start of a viral infection can be treated using remedies such as echinacea (*Echinacea* spp.), licorice (*Glycyrrhiza glabra*), and sage (*Salvia officinalis*). Take tea or diluted tincture of one or more of these remedies, first as a gargle, then swallow. Continue taking three times a day until symptoms have cleared. If symptoms deteriorate sharply or there is no improvement after five days, seek professional advice.

CHRONIC PROBLEMS

Problems that have lingered for months or even years, such as acid indigestion, osteoarthritis, and fungal skin infections, can be successfully relieved or improved with herbal remedies, although long-term treatment may be required (a rule of thumb used by herbal practitioners is one month's treatment for every year the condition has been present). Taking a remedy regularly is likely to prove more effective than occasional dosing when symptoms flare. That being said, there is nothing wrong in using herbal remedies for symptomatic relief.

APPLYING SAGE
Fresh sage (*Salvia officinalis*) leaves are antiseptic and can be rubbed on insect bites and stings.

Example Acid indigestion can be relieved (and hopefully reversed) by taking meadowsweet (*Filipendula ulmaria*) tea or tincture after meals for several months. Other remedies such as slippery elm (*Ulmus fulva*) and chamomile (*Chamomilla recutita*) may also prove helpful, as will attention to diet.

PREVENTING ILLNESS

Taken long-term, many herbal remedies have been shown to have a potent ability to prevent illness or deterioration in existing symptoms. Indeed, some would argue that working on the basis that prevention is the best medicine is the way to use herbal remedies. The difficulty with a preventive approach of course is that, if successful, one does not see results. Such an approach nevertheless comes close to the ancient Chinese emperor's practice of paying his doctors only as long as he remained well. As a result it was always in his doctors' interest to act preventatively rather than once illness had taken hold.

MEADOWSWEET
Meadowsweet tea or tincture is commonly taken to relieve digestive problems such as acidity, indigestion, and diarrhea.

Example Millions of people take ginkgo (*Ginkgo biloba*) on a daily basis in order to maintain healthy blood flow to the brain and limbs and to prevent dementia, both uses that are strongly supported by clinical research. The herb's notable antioxidant activity also helps prevent inflammation and allergy.

ENHANCING HEALTH

Herbs can prove extremely helpful in promoting mental and physical performance, particularly where constitutional weaknesses exist. Whether taken by students studying for exams or athletes preparing for an event (who should remember that herbal remedies may test positive in drug testing), remedies with tonic and adaptogenic properties support endurance and the ability to cope with stress. Night shift workers, people

putting in long hours or tolerating extreme conditions in the workplace, and those suffering from long-term stress may all benefit from such remedies.

Example For exams and interviews, mental focus and vitality can be enhanced with herbs such as rosemary (*Rosmarinus officinalis*) and schisandra (*Schisandra chinensis*)— but note that when taking these herbs it is important to try them out first, before the exam or interview. Similarly, people working long hours or nights can benefit from remedies such as Siberian ginseng (*Eleutherococcus senticosus*) or golden root (*Rhodiola rosea*) to improve their stamina and work rate.

SCHISANDRA
A Chinese tonic herb, schisandra is commonly taken to improve liver metabolism and enhance mental stamina and performance.

ARE HERBAL REMEDIES SAFE?

With a few exceptions, all of the herbal remedies in this book are recognized as safe for home use. The few that are not, such as lobelia (*Lobelia inflata*), are commonly included in manufactured herbal products and are safe when taken as instructed.

All of the remedies listed have some evidence of effectiveness, although this varies greatly from plant to plant. The ability of ginkgo (*Ginkgo biloba*) to improve memory and prevent dementia is strongly supported by research evidence. On the other hand, the use of chickweed (*Stellaria media*) to soothe itchy skin and eczema has never been researched, and rests upon traditional knowledge and direct experience.

The safety of herbal remedies, and their effectiveness as medicines, is not necessarily easy to establish. By and large, knowledge about how herbs work comes from:
• Use as food or a food supplement.
• Traditional knowledge of use as a medicine.

• The experience of herbal practitioners.
• Scientific research.

NUTRITION

Remedies such as garlic (*Allium sativum*), lemon (*Citrus limon*), oats (*Avena sativa*), and soy (*Glycine max*) form a regular part of many people's diets, and are therefore used as both food and medicine. Long-term food use confirms that the remedy is safe to take as a medicine, although it tells one little about its effectiveness in this respect. Some herbal remedies contain significant levels of nutrients and are taken as nutritional supplements, for example, kelp (*Fucus vesiculosis*). Such use comes from scientific investigation of the plant's constituents.

KNOWLEDGE

The strength of traditional medicinal systems such as Ayurvedic (India/Sri Lanka), Chinese, and Western herbal medicine lies in the fact that knowledge and experience of remedies has been built up over thousands of years, constituting what has been described as the longest-ever clinical trial. Put to the test of time, it is argued, few herbs that are harmful or ineffective will remain in popular

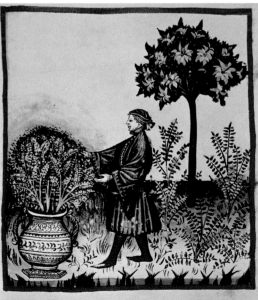

Oʒimuin auruií.ꝓ pſo.caꞇa in .t. ſic.in ꝑ. Qecꞇo bn̄ aꞇouſeꝛ. ꝑꞇiꞁichꞇ.eꞇ iba ſtn̄giꞇ. ſue ꞇaueꞇ uenꞇꞇm̄.Tooun̄iuin.obeꞇnebꞋꞇ uꞇꞇiu.Ⱪ emoꞒo naꞇn̄in.äi poꞇꞃulꞇei.Qø gn̄a꞉ꞇ bumoꞇe; aciꞇluin.ꞇ inꝼꞇꞇauuuin.ꞎuen̄iꞇ꞉ ꞓꞃiꞑ.ſeibꞓ.bꞇeme꞉ꞇ ſeꝑꞇꞃuꞇꝺnꞇꞇꞇbꞇ.

AN ANCIENT TRADITION
Effective herbal remedies such as licorice (*Glycyrrhiza glabra*) have been grown and used as medicines for thousands of years.

use—only those found to be safe and effective will retain their place. Longstanding use of a herbal remedy can therefore be seen as a strong indicator of safety and usefulness, although it is *not* a guarantee.

EXPERIENCE

Trained herbal practitioners develop a practical, subtle understanding of how best to apply herbal medicines and are watchful for signs of side effects. They are able to select those remedies most likely to help a patient. The collective experience of herbal practitioners—for example, caution in giving devil's claw (*Harpagophytum procumbens*) to patients with acid indigestion—can give important pointers to the safety and effectiveness of remedies.

RESEARCH

Scientific investigation into a medicinal plant spans a multitude of different types of research which add, like pieces in a jigsaw puzzle, to the overall picture. Researchers can investigate:
• The chemistry of the plant—its constituents and their actions.
• The whole plant—parts used, actions, uses, safety issues, and so forth.
• Processing—how to extract and process the remedy.
• Clinical trials—the therapeutic use of a plant extract, including dosage levels, safety, and evidence of effectiveness.
On one level, the chemistry of the plant, or phytochemistry, underpins all aspects of herbal research. If you know the key chemical constituents of a plant, you can make a reasonable guess about its level of safety and value as a medicine: caffeine is a key constituent in coffee (*Coffea arabica*), cola, guarana (*Paulinia cupana*), mate (*Ilex paraguariensis*), and tea (*Camellia sinensis*). Its stimulant activity forms part of the action of each plant.

Yet, each plant also has its own unique activity and character. The natural complex of constituents found

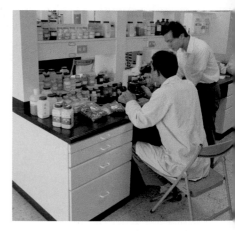

MODERN METHODS
Scientific research starts by analyzing the chemistry of the plant. Scientists can then investigate how key active components influence its medicinal activity.

within a herbal remedy—the "whole"—is more than its key active constituents—"the sum of its parts." This interplay or synergy between different constituents is often a factor in the safety and effectiveness of an herbal medicine (see also Types of herbal remedy, pp.30–33).

Good clinical trials compare the safety and efficacy of an herbal medicine against another medicine or a placebo (a dummy product). Data collected from these trials provides the strongest evidence of just how safe or effective an herbal remedy is.

NEW USE FOR CINNAMON

The marriage between traditional knowledge and scientific research can lead to exciting new insights into the use of herbal remedies. Cinnamon (*Cinnamomum verum*) is a good example. While it is used in Asian traditional medicine for colds, flu, and digestive problems, recent investigations indicate that it has a potent stabilizing effect on blood sugar levels, helping to slow or prevent the onset of diabetes. It is also active against *Helicobacter pylori*, a bacterium commonly linked with stomach ulcers.

CINNAMON BARK

HOW REMEDIES WORK

Around the world, people's knowledge of how herbal medicines work varies widely. In many traditional societies, spirits are thought to be responsible for a plant's activity, while in others the appearance and structure of a plant—its "signature"—indicates its use as a medicine.

ANIMAL MAGIC

Observation of how animals use medicinal plants has undoubtedly been a key factor behind the traditional use of many plants, and is now itself the subject of scientific study. Around the world, animals from bears to snakes have been observed eating plants with specific medicinal activity only at those times when they are in need of them. Animals may also acquire a taste for plants that have general effects. The stimulant activity of coffee (*Coffea arabica*) was reputedly discovered after goatherds noted the frisky behavior of goats feeding on the bush's red berries!

HOW PLANTS WORK

Many people, including herbal practitioners, believe that medicinal plants work in part on an energetic level, each plant having a distinct vitality, reflecting perhaps some kind of electromagnetic force. Understanding the vitality, or vital force, of a remedy gives clues that can be used to refine its use as a medicine, in particular helping to match specific remedies with the needs of individual patients. That being said, scientific research provides the greatest certainty that a remedy is safe to use and has a reasonable chance of being effective. Scientific study of medicinal plants and their chemical constituents underpins our understanding of how herbal remedies work, and provides precise information on a plant's therapeutic activity and potential use as a medicine.

NATURE'S MEDICINE
Bears are known to seek out and eat large quantities of antioxidant-rich roots and berries shortly before going into hibernation.

ACTIVE CONSTITUENTS

The main types of active constituent found in herbal remedies are listed below. Medicinal plants typically contain hundreds of different constituents with only a small proportion having direct therapeutic activity. As a rule, if you know a plant's active constituents you can broadly predict its medicinal effects, for example linden flowers (*Tilia* spp.) contain a volatile oil with sedative activity, flavonoids, mucilage, and phenols. These constituents correlate with linden flower's standard use as a remedy: to aid sleep and relaxation, relieve headache and fever, and lower blood pressure and support the circulation.

CONSTITUENT	COMMON MEDICINAL ACTIVITY	EXAMPLES
Phenols	Often have anti-inflammatory, antiseptic, and antioxidant properties	Salicylic acid, found in willow bark (*Salix alba*)
Volatile oils	Complex mixtures of plant compounds with a wide range of actions, including stimulant, sedative, anti-inflammatory, and insecticidal properties	Essential oil of tea tree (*Melaleuca alternifolia*)
Flavonoids	Often pigments with a yellow or white color; many are strongly antioxidant and benefit the circulation, some are estrogenic	Rutin, found in lemon (*Citrus limon*) pith and peel
Tannins	Have astringent, binding (or tanning) action; often with potent antioxidant and anti-inflammatory properties	Catechins, found in witch hazel (*Hamamelis virginiana*)
Coumarins	Often have blood-thinning or antispasmodic properties	Aesculin, found in horse chestnut seed (*Aesculus hippocastanum*)
Saponins	Key medicinal compounds similar in structure to the body's own hormones, often having hormonal or anti inflammatory activity	Dioscin, found in Mexican wild yam (*Dioscorea villosa*)
Anthraquinones	Constituents that at the right dosage act as laxatives	Sennosides, found in senna (*Cassia* spp.)
Cardiac glycosides	Powerful compounds that act on the heart, often toxic	Digitoxin, found in foxglove (*Digitalis purpurea*)
Cyanogenic glycosides	Compounds that contain cyanide; at low doses valuable as sedatives and relaxants	Sambunigrin, found in elder leaves (*Sambucus nigra*)
Polysaccharides	Large molecules that typically have a demulcent/soothing effect on mucous membranes	Mucilage, found in slippery elm (*Ulmus fulva*)
Bitters	Strongly bitter-tasting compounds that stimulate appetite and digestive function and slow the heart	Amarogentin, found in gentian (*Gentiana lutea*)
Alkaloids	A diverse group of compounds, some with very potent activity as medicines, for example morphine	Isoquinoline alkaoids, found in Californian poppy (*Eschscholzia californica*)

LEMON

HORSE CHESTNUT

FOXGLOVE

Medicinal plants also contain nutrients, vitamins, and minerals. In a few cases, for example alfalfa (*Medicago sativa*) and kelp (*Fucus* spp.), vitamin and mineral levels are significant, although in most cases only trace levels are present.

AROUND THE WORLD

Looked at from a global perspective, herbal medicine is humanity's most important resource for treating and relieving illness. Although conventional biochemical medicine provides the bulk of medical treatment in Western countries, this is far from the case elsewhere.

In China and India in particular, traditional medicine is as popular as its conventional counterpart, and the vast majority of remedies used are herbal. In China, people choose whether to receive traditional or biochemical treatment, although in practice biochemical medicine is recommended for acute and life-threatening illness, and herbal medicine for chronic, long-term illness.

RESEARCHING THE HERBS

The sheer scale of traditional Chinese medicine means that research and development in China has brought new insights into herbal remedies. Clinical research in Shanghai into Chinese wormwood (*Artemisia annua*)—a traditional Chinese remedy for malaria that grows in temperate regions around the world—led to the discovery that it was a highly effective treatment for malaria. The herb, and in particular its key active constituent, artemisinin, is at present the only certain treatment for severe malarial illness.

In many parts of the world, particularly Africa, the vast majority of medicines are herbal. In Ghana, over 80 percent of medicines used are herbal, most of which are prepared from native West African medicinal plants. Paralleling developments elsewhere in the world, moves are afoot to produce an African Pharmacopoeia that will provide scientific and medical data on 53 key African medicinal

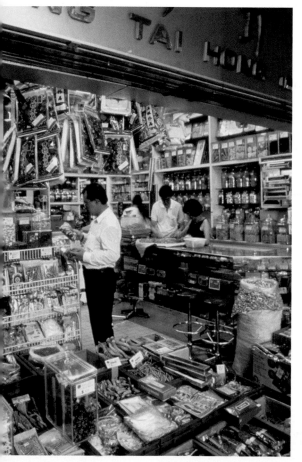

CHINESE MEDICINE
Traditional Chinese medicine centers and herb suppliers are now a common sight in shopping centers all over the world. In China, herbal remedies remain the preferred form of self-treatment for everyday health problems such as upset stomach.

plants, including remedies such as *Withania somnifera*.

Even in Western countries, a sizeable minority of medicines used are herbal. About 25 percent of the medicines used in the British National Health Service are herbal in origin, while in Germany 90 percent of doctors routinely prescribe herbal medicines to their patients, hawthorn (*Crataegus* spp.) and saw palmetto (*Serenoa serrulata*) being common examples.

Germany is a world center for research into herbal or phyto-medicines, and German research from the 1940s onward has been responsible for establishing the safety and effectiveness of many popular over-the-counter remedies like ginkgo (*Ginkgo biloba*). Worldwide, research into herbal medicines is expanding at an unprecedented rate. Many countries have set up and support national research centers.

OVER THE COUNTER

Sales of over-the-counter herbal remedies grew phenomenally in the 1990s and have since leveled off. The top 10 individual best sellers in the

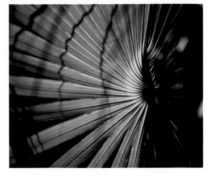

SAW PALMETTO
In Europe, saw palmetto is one of several herbal medicines routinely prescribed by doctors to treat symptoms resulting from an enlarged prostate.

US in 2005 are listed in the box below. Most of these individual remedies are also global best sellers, although products combining several different herbal remedies are becoming increasingly popular.

Recent legislation in Australia and in the European Union has established quality standards and labeling requirements for herbal remedies that should guarantee the quality of products sold in health food stores and pharmacies. The legislation may have less impact on Internet or mail-order sales. In the US, herbal remedies are generally classified as food supplements and are marketed under regulations governing food rather than medicines.

HERBAL PRACTITIONERS

As herbal medicine has grown in popularity, so has the need for trained practitioners who are able to assess a patient's needs and provide sound advice and treatment. In Western countries such as the US, Australia, Ireland, and the UK, university training for herbal practitioners and naturopaths has become the norm; for these degree courses, practitioners are trained in both medical and herbal sciences. In China and India, universities teaching traditional medicine train practitioners to a standard equivalent to that of conventional medical practitioners.

TOP TEN OVER-THE-COUNTER REMEDIES

The following ten herbs were the best sellers in the US in 2005:

1. Garlic (*Allium sativum*)
2. Echinacea (*Echinacea* spp.)
3. Saw palmetto (*Serenoa serrulata*)
4. Ginkgo (*Ginkgo biloba*)
5. Cranberry (*Vaccinium macrocarpon*)
6. Soy (*Glycine max*)
7. Ginseng (*Panax ginseng*)
8. Black cohosh (*Cimicifuga racemosa*)
9. St. John's wort (*Hypericum perforatum*)
10. Milk thistle (*Silybum marianum*)

SOURCE HerbalGram 2006 (www.herbalgram.com)

ECHINACEA

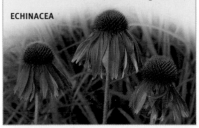

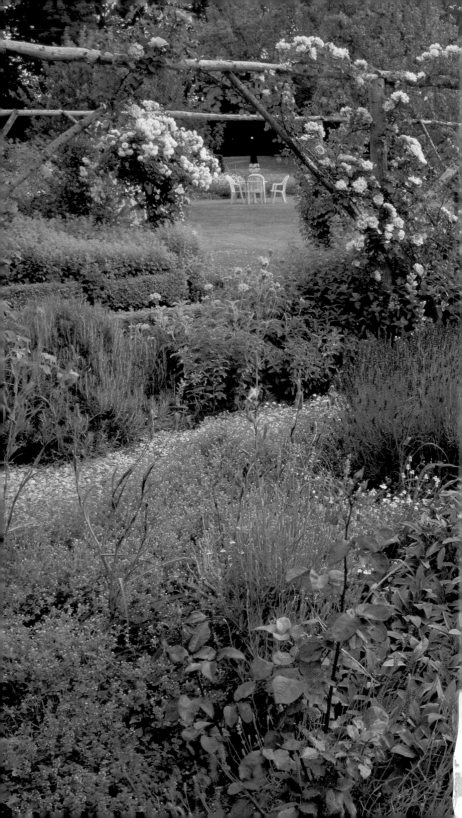

USING HERBAL REMEDIES

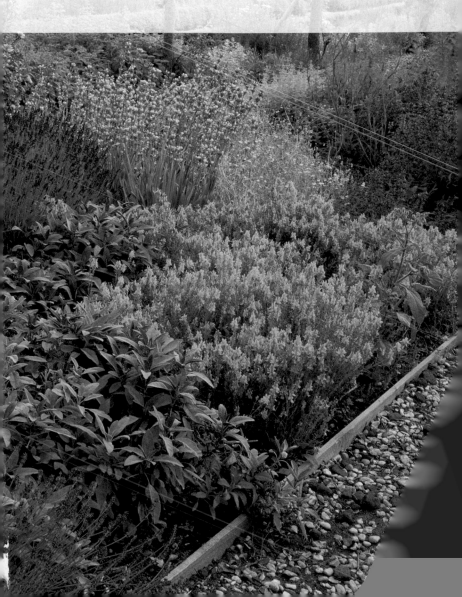

MAKING HERBAL MEDICINES

The journey from hedgerow, garden, or medicinal plant farm to the finished herbal product takes many different forms. Wherever they are grown, however, medicinal plants need to be harvested and processed appropriately to achieve good-quality results and effective remedies.

Wild-crafting and cultivation

Many medicinal plants are still regularly picked from the wild— a process known as wild-crafting. Even in the developed world, herbs such as elder flowers and berries (*Sambucus nigra*), found in hedgerows and roadsides throughout the US and Europe, are wild-crafted both on a commercial basis and locally, to make herbal medicines and medicinal wines.

In the developing world, herbs are as often wild-crafted as cultivated. In some cases, for example in some African countries, nearly 90 percent of herbal medicines used are gathered from the wild. Such a dependence on wild-crafting can threaten the survival of

important medicinal plant species, especially if roots or bark are the main part of the plant used.

However, the main threat comes from commercial wild-crafting, where plants are gathered as a cash crop for export rather than for use locally as medicines. There are many examples of medicinal plants being pushed close to the point of extinction in this way— goldenseal (*Hydrastis canadensis*) in North America and arnica (*Arnica montana*) in

ENDANGERED SPECIES
The survival of many medicinal plants is threatened in the wild. Buy organic or conservation-grade products wherever possible.

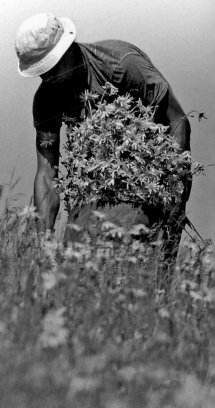

Europe are threatened species that are now being extensively cultivated. Until recently, echinacea (*Echinacea* spp.) was a common wild plant in its native North America; due to excessive wild-crafting, it is now rare to find it in the wild.

The Convention on International Trade in Endangered Species of Wild Flora and Fauna (CITES) accord helps prevent trade in endangered plant species, and by and large the needs of economics and conservation point the same way; cultivation makes better sense. Common medicinal plants such as German chamomile (*Chamomilla recutita*) are grown on a large scale in places as far afield as Egypt and Argentina. Demand for ginkgo (*Ginkgo*

biloba) has led to large plantations now found in countries such as France and the USA, where the leaves are harvested by agricultural machinery. As demand for herbal medicine grows, large-scale cultivation is more economically viable.

Organically grown medicinal plants are to be preferred over conventionally grown ones. Being produced without chemical interference, they develop naturally and absorb nutrients from the soil. They should also be relatively free from inorganic fertilizers, pesticides, and pollutants. Organic certification provides some evidence that a plant meets certain quality standards and has been cultivated or wild-crafted in an ecologically sensitive manner.

Harvesting and drying

Whatever the size of the crop, the same basic rules apply. Although drying sheds and dehumidifiers are used industrially, a warm, well-ventilated drying rack such as an airing cabinet or a low-heated oven with the door open will suffice. Collect only plant material that you will be able to use or dry at once.

HARVESTING HERBS

- Try to harvest on a sunny, dry morning after the dew has evaporated.
- Ensure that you are picking the right plant, and the right part of it; using the wrong part may be dangerous.
- Use a sharp knife or scissors; cut perennials to encourage regrowth.
- Do not pick plants with blight or insect damage, nor plants growing in a polluted area.
- Plants are generally best harvested in the following stages: flowers, when just opening; leaves, when fully open; fruits, berries, and seeds, when ripe; whole plants, when mature.

DRYING

- Drying is best done in a shaded, well-ventilated area. Racks within a drying frame or airing cabinet are good, especially for leaves, flowers, roots, and bark, but whole plants can be hung up from a shaded line. Fresh plant material can be chopped and laid out on brown paper to dry; do not use newsprint—the inks are toxic.
- Discard poorly dried plant material, for example where the leaves are discolored or where they show signs of fungal infection.
- Once dry, chop or break up the herb material into small pieces suitable for storage in labeled, sterilized glass jars or brown paper bags.

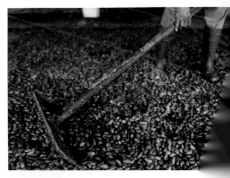

DRIED HERBS
Careful, unrushed drying, no matter how large or small the scale, is a key element in the production good-quality herb material.

Industrial processing

Although many people's image of herbal medicine involves pans of bubbling liquids and strange-smelling bottles, the truth is that in many parts of the world, herbal products—tablets and capsules especially—are likely to be produced in a setting as far away from the kitchen countertop as possible. A large part of the herbal medicine industry is perhaps more accurately known as the phyto-pharmaceutical industry, with multimillion dollar, high-tech, hermetically sealed factories. Many larger herb growers and phyto-pharmaceutical manufacturers are in fact owned by mainstream pharmaceutical companies. Enter one of the large phyto-pharmaceutical manufacturing sites and you will only find evidence of the herbal origin of its products in the Goods Inward section!

Remedies produced on an industrial scale to good manufacturing practice (GMP) standards are likely to be of good quality, and might be expected to be better than those produced in a more traditional, low-tech manner. However, much as is the case with small-scale, high-quality wine production, small-scale herb manufacturers often manage to produce plant material and herbal remedies of a distinctly higher quality than industrially produced over-the-counter remedies. That being said, GMP gives the buyer assurance that over-the-counter products should consistently meet acceptable quality standards.

CAPSULES AND TABLETS

Most capsules and tablets are industrially produced. Some are made with finely powdered herb material, though many are manufactured from or dry extracts. Various liquid solvents are used to dissolve the main active constituents found in the plant. These are then evaporated off, leaving a soft extract that contains about 20–30 percent water. Dry extracts are easily powdered and typically contain no more than 5 percent water. These extracts are then prepared as tablets, for example, to provide a uniform dose.

STANDARDIZED EXTRACTS

Standardized dried herb material or extracts are herbal products—typically capsules, tablets, and tinctures—that contain a minimum level of one or more key constituents. Using sensitive scientific measuring equipment, for example high-performance liquid chromatography (HPLC), batches of herb material are tested to establish levels of these constituents. Batches that meet the required levels of a given constituent are termed "standardized." Ginkgo (*Ginkgo biloba*), standardized on its flavone glycoside content, and milk thistle (*Silybum marianum*), standardized on its silymarin content, are common examples.

Some herbs are standardized on two different constituents: in the case of St. John's wort (*Hypericum perforatum*), some products are standardized on its hypericin content, some on its hyperforin content, and some on both!

Most people would agree that this kind of quality control is valuable, especially in over-the-counter remedies. However, a more sophisticated method looks at the chemical fingerprint of the plant—the overall pattern of constituents extracted—that reflects the plant's natural complexity, sometimes referred to as a "full spectrum" of ingredients. Many people argue that this approach more accurately reflects herbal quality: it is the complex mix of constituents in a plant, not just one or

GINKGO TABLETS

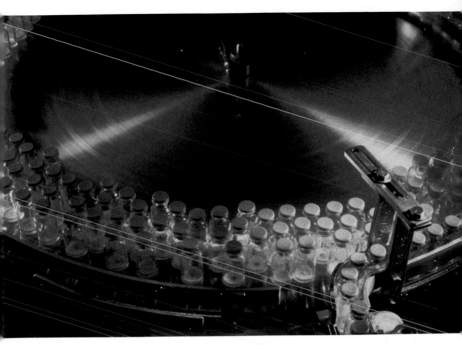

INDUSTRIAL PRODUCTION
Industrially produced herbal remedies made to GMP standards should consistently be of good quality, and can be purchased with confidence over the counter.

two isolated constituents, that produces its medicinal benefit. At least five different processes have been identified that contribute to the antidepressant activity of St. John's wort, for example. For this reason, herbal practitioners typically stock and dispense dried herbs and tinctures produced by small-scale manufacturers who use this "full spectrum" method of quality control.

PURIFIED EXTRACTS

A strong case can be made that standardized extracts that are purified—where levels of some constituents are enhanced at the expense of others—are not herbal remedies at all, but part-herbal, part-chemical medicines. Purified extracts are often highly concentrated—indeed, selected constituents can be so highly concentrated, by up to 2000-fold, that few other plant chemicals will be present. Such products may be

valuable, but they cannot fairly claim to be herbal medicines. Red clover (*Trifolium pratense*) isoflavone extracts, and some aloe vera (*Aloe vera*) products, are examples of this type of process.

When buying herbal remedies, look at the label for information about standardization and refer to What the label should tell you on pp.50–51.

SKIN CREAMS
Good-quality herbal skin creams undergo the same quality-control procedures as capsules, tablets, or tinctures.

TYPES OF HERBAL REMEDY

Herbal remedies are prepared and used in many different ways, and it can often be hard to decide which form of remedy to select. The following section gives details of the main types of herbal preparation available, along with a summary of their pros and cons.

Herbal remedies can be made in a number of different ways, each method having its own specific advantages and disadvantages. Many preparations, for example teas and tinctures, are traditional and have been used to make medicines for thousands of years; no specialized equipment is required to make them. Others, however, require modern pharmaceutical methods of extraction, and use a wide range of solvents and processes. Such extracts are most frequently made into tablets and capsules.

EXTRACTING THE ACTIVE

Though it is not commonly recognized, the processes used to make a medicine directly influence its effect on the body. For example, ginger root (*Zingiber officinalis*) can be eaten fresh or dried in food, taken as a powder or capsule, made into a tea or tincture, or processed to produce a concentrated extract. In small but nonetheless significant ways, each process extracts a different cross-section of chemicals within the plant, known as "the active." Ginger contains antiseptic resins that are poorly soluble in water, so ginger tea contains almost no resins; however, a ginger tincture made with 90 percent alcohol (ethanol) extracts them well, thus having a greater antiseptic activity.

In day-to-day life, roughly the same applies to coffee. Espresso machines were designed to extract maximum

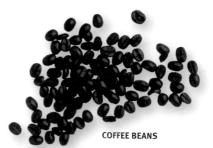

COFFEE BEANS

flavor and, contrary to popular belief, relatively low levels of caffeine. In contrast, coffee percolators extract far higher levels of caffeine while much of the finer flavor is destroyed by the continued heating. (Percolated coffee is not thought to be a healthy way to drink coffee.)

The following are the most frequently used types of herbal preparation. Details on making remedies are given in The home herbal on pp.36–37. For dosage advice, see pp.44–45.

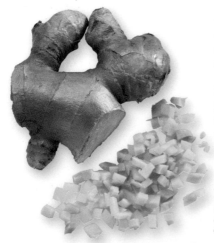

GINGER
Fresh and dried ginger root are seen as distinct remedies in Chinese herbal medicine. As the root dries, new compounds are formed and some of the essential oil in the fresh root evaporates.

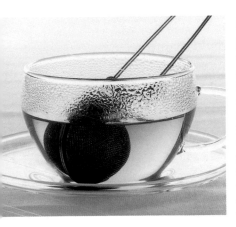

HERBAL INFUSIONS
Brewing tea bags or an infuser in an open cup is fine for nonaromatic herbs. Brew herbs that contain essential oils in a teapot.

TEAS/INFUSIONS

Teas, or infusions, are the simplest way to make an herbal remedy, using the more delicate aerial (above-ground) parts of a plant—especially fresh or dried leaves and flowers. Teas are good for extracting water-soluble constituents such as flavonoids, for example in hawthorn leaves (*Crataegus* spp.), and essential oils, for example in peppermint (*Mentha × piperita*). Use a glass or ceramic (not metal) pot or cup with a lid to infuse the herb. Loose herbs are generally better than teabags— it can be stirred and dispersed throughout the teapot or cup, improving extraction. Brew for 10 minutes then strain.

Pros Quick and easy to make; several herbs can be combined; fresh or dried herb material can be used; can be drunk, used as a mouthwash or gargle, applied as a lotion, hair rinse, and so forth; being diluted in water, is fairly easily absorbed.

Cons Must be used quickly (maximum 24 hours, refrigerated); only water-soluble constituents extracted; taste can be unpleasant; a relatively large amount of liquid needs to be consumed.

DECOCTIONS

Decoctions are the most straightforward way to prepare tougher plant parts such as bark, berries, and roots. Chopped fresh or dried material is simmered in water for about 20 minutes. The resulting liquid is strained and drunk. Decoctions are good for extracting water-soluble constituents such as tannins, for example in witch hazel bark (*Hamamelis virginiana*). Like infusions, they have long traditional use and are still the main method of preparation used in traditional Chinese medicine.

Pros Can use fresh or dried herb material; several herbs can be combined; can be drunk, used as a mouthwash or gargle, applied as a lotion, and so forth; being diluted in water, fairly easily absorbed.

Cons Take a little time to make; must be consumed quickly (maximum 48 hours, refrigerated); taste can be very unpleasant.

DECOCTION OF SCHISANDRA

JUICES

Juices can be bought or made at home. High-powered juice extractors are better than standard fruit and vegetable juicers. When properly prepared, juices contain a wide range of constituents, including enzymes that are lost when the plant is dried. Use organic produce as far as possible.

Pros Relatively easy to make; 100 percent natural product with high enzyme and micro-nutrient content; easily absorbed and aid digestive function.

Cons Must be kept refrigerated and, if bottled, consumed within 10 days; bes not combined with other herbs; taste can be unpleasant.

TINCTURES

Tinctures are made by macerating (soaking) chopped herb material from any part of the plant in an alcohol solution, typically 45 percent alcohol to 55 percent water. The proportion of alcohol used varies from 25 percent to 90 percent, depending upon the active constituents to be extracted. Sometimes vinegar or glycerol is used instead of alcohol. Tinctures are relatively easily made and keep well, for three years or more. By using an alcohol and water mix both water-soluble and non-water-soluble constituents can be extracted, leading to a more concentrated product than is possible with teas or decoctions. The ratio of herb material to water and alcohol determines the strength of the tincture. An appropriate strength for most commonly available tinctures is 1 part herb material to 3 parts water and alcohol.

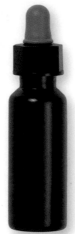

TINCTURE

Pros Long shelf life; different tinctures easily combined together; wide range of constituents extracted; small amounts effective; very easily absorbed.

Cons Takes several days to produce but can be easily purchased; can taste very unpleasant; contains alcohol (sometimes at high levels).

SYRUPS

yrups are usually made by adding
·refined sugar or honey to infusions
·decoctions at a ratio of 1:1 (half
half). Their sweetness can mask

unpalatable herbs. The sugars help soothe irritation within the throat and chest, and syrups are classically used as cough mixtures. Syrups, linctuses, and cordials can be bought over the counter or made at home.

Pros Fairly long shelf life; sweet-tasting and can be combined with unpleasant-tasting remedies; good for coughs.

Cons Large amounts of sugar; limited applications.

CAPSULES

Capsules generally contain dried powdered herb material or soft or dry concentrated extracts. Good-quality capsules are densely packed so that air cannot circulate through the powder. Vegetarian or non-vegetarian gelatine capsules (size 00) can be purchased for filling at home. Sealed capsules containing oils or concentrated soft or dry extracts are similar in action to tablets (see below) but usually contain fewer binding agents and additives.

Pros Convenient to take, and with little taste; clearly defined dose; often standardized.

Cons Cannot be blended like tinctures; powders can occasionally be irritant; may be excessively concentrated.

GARLIC CAPSULES

TABLETS

Tablets can be made by simply compressing dried herb material or a dry extract into tablet form, though usually herb material is combined with excipients (binding agents and additives) that maintain the tablet's shape and structure but dissolve in the stomach or intestines. Regrettably, artificial sweeteners and colors are often used in tablet formulation, so read the label.

Pros Convenient and concentrated; clearly defined dose; often standardized; little taste.

Cons May dissolve poorly in the digestive tract; may be excessively concentrated; cannot be blended like tinctures.

BOSWELLIA TABLETS

FIXED OILS

Unlike essential oils, fixed oils are made by soaking herb material in a vegetable oil, such as sunflower. Fixed oils are typically made with herbs that have wound-healing properties, for example marigold (*Calendula officinalis*), and can be applied neat to minor cuts, grazes, sprains, and so forth. They can also be used in creams and ointments.

Pros Easily massaged into the skin: blend well with essential oils.

Cons Often greasy—ointments or creams may be better.

FREEZE-DRIED EXTRACTS

Used increasingly in traditional Chinese medicine, freeze-dried extracts are made using a process similar to instant coffee. They have the full range of constituents found in the herb or herb formula.

Pros Convenient; clearly defined dose; often standardized.

Cons Expensive; not readily available.

POWDERS

Used traditionally in Ayurvedic medicine, powders are easy to take. They tend to deteriorate quicker than normal dried herb material.

Pros Easy to take.

Cons May taste unpleasant; need to be carefully stored.

MYRRH POWDER

OINTMENTS AND CREAMS

Ointments are made using oils and fats, and usually contain no water. Being oily they form a waterproof, protective surface on the skin and are most useful in conditions such as hemorrhoids and diaper rash. Creams are made by emulsifying oils and water in an emulsion, much as in mayonnaise. They are cooling and moisten the skin, and are used to soothe sore and inflamed skin conditions. Avoid applying ointments and creams to open wounds.

Pros Formulated for the skin.

Cons May contain artificial preservatives and stabilizers.

ESSENTIAL OILS

Essential oils are mostly produced by distilling flowers, leaves, and so forth and collecting the resulting oil – the plant's "essence." Being very concentrated, they must be used with care. Typically, they are blended in a carrier oil such as grapeseed oil at a *maximum* 5 percent dilution, for example 1ml of essential oil in 20ml of carrier oil, or 5 drops in a teaspoon of carrier oil. Essential oils should not be taken internally, unless on the instruction of a suitably qualified doctor, medical herbalist, or naturopath.

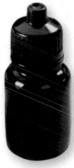

LAVENDER ESSENTIAL OIL

Pros Highly concentrate[d?] pleasant aroma; can be used diluted on skin o[r] dispersed in air by b[urning].

Cons Can occasion[ally] irritation or allergic reactions.

HERBAL REMEDIES AT HOME

Making simple herbal preparations is easy provided you follow a few straightforward rules—the most important being to start with correctly identified herb material. The dosages given below apply to most (but not all) commonly available herbal remedies—see pp.44–45.

PREPARING A HERBAL TEA

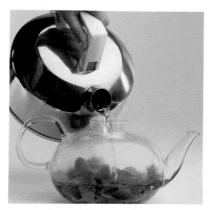
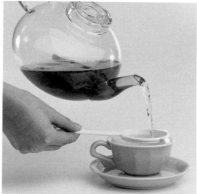

1 Add 1 heaped teaspoonful of fresh or 1 level teaspoonful of dried herb material (leaves, flowers) to a teapot. Pour in a cupful of boiling water.

2 Stir, cover, and let stand for 10 minutes. Strain, add honey if desired, and drink.

PREPARING A DECOCTION

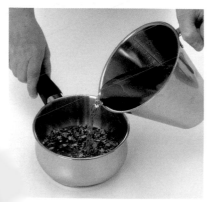
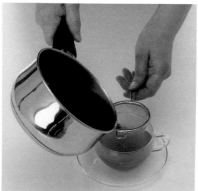

1 heaped teaspoonful of fresh or erb material (bark, berries, root) in a nonaluminum saucepan. ups of water and gently bring immer for approximately

2 Remove from the heat and carefully strain into a cup or other container. Add honey if desired and drink. Larger quantities can be prepared if required, for example 1oz (25g) herb material to ¼ cup water.

PREPARING A TINCTURE

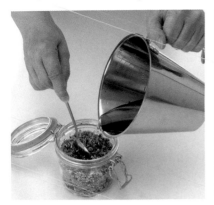

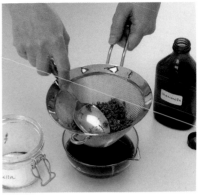

1 A standard tincture is made using 1 part dried herb material to 3 parts alcohol solution. Place the chopped herb material—root, leaf, flower, or fruit—in a clean, preferably sterilized, glass jar or pan and stir in the required amount of alcohol. For each 4oz (100g) of dried herb material, add 1 cup of alcohol solution (for strength see box shown right). Stir well, make sure that herb material is fully covered, close lid, and label clearly.

2 Stir or shake the contents thoroughly for a few minutes each day, for 10 days. Strain into a sterilized glass bottle, seal with a cap, and label.

ALCOHOL SOLUTION

For tinctures, use organic vodka or other good-quality spirit of similar strength. Fresh plant materials require a 40 percent alcohol solution. Dried plant material can be made with lower-strength alcohol, typically 25 percent. Below 20 percent, alcohol solution tinctures may decay.

STORING HERBAL MATERIAL AT HOME

Dried herb material is best stored in glass jars. Jars should be clean and dry, and preferably sterilized. Fill the jar close to the top with herb material and close the lid firmly.

For short-term storage (a few months) dried herb material can be kept in clean brown paper bags, folded over and secured with a rubber band. Clearly label the jar or bag with the following information:

● Name, and part, of plant

● Date of harvesting.

● Keep in a cool, dry, dark place, away from heat and direct sunlight. Keep out of reach of children and animals.

● Dried herbs should be used within 12 months of harvesting. Tinctures can remain effective for 3 years or more. Capsules and tablets should have a "Use by" date on the container.

● Dried herb material that changes color due to damp or fungal infection, or has mites (insect infestation), should not be used. Put it in the garden compost or place in a sealed plastic bag in a waste bin.

THE HOME HERBAL

Herbal remedies can prove highly effective in treating minor health and first aid problems. Cuts, scrapes, headaches, digestive upsets, and so on can be dealt with effectively using just a few herbal products. Keeping a range of remedies available makes good sense.

First aid kit

Selecting herbal remedies to complement a standard first aid kit containing standard items such as adhesive bandages and scissors can be an enjoyable activity. The 10 remedies shown below are readily available in natural pharmacies and health food stores and are useful to have at home for minor domestic emergencies. For details of their uses and applications, see the relevant entry in the A–Z section on pages 52–255.

Note Creams and ointments should not be put on open wounds: use water, aloe vera (*Aloe vera*), or witch hazel (*Hamamelis virginiana*) water to wash cuts and scrapes, and then bathe with diluted echinacea (*Echinacea* spp.) or myrrh (*Commiphora molmol*) tincture. Warning! This will disinfect the area but will sting painfully for a short time. Burns should be held under cold water for at least 10 minutes before applying aloe vera or lavender (*Lavendula* spp.) essential oil.

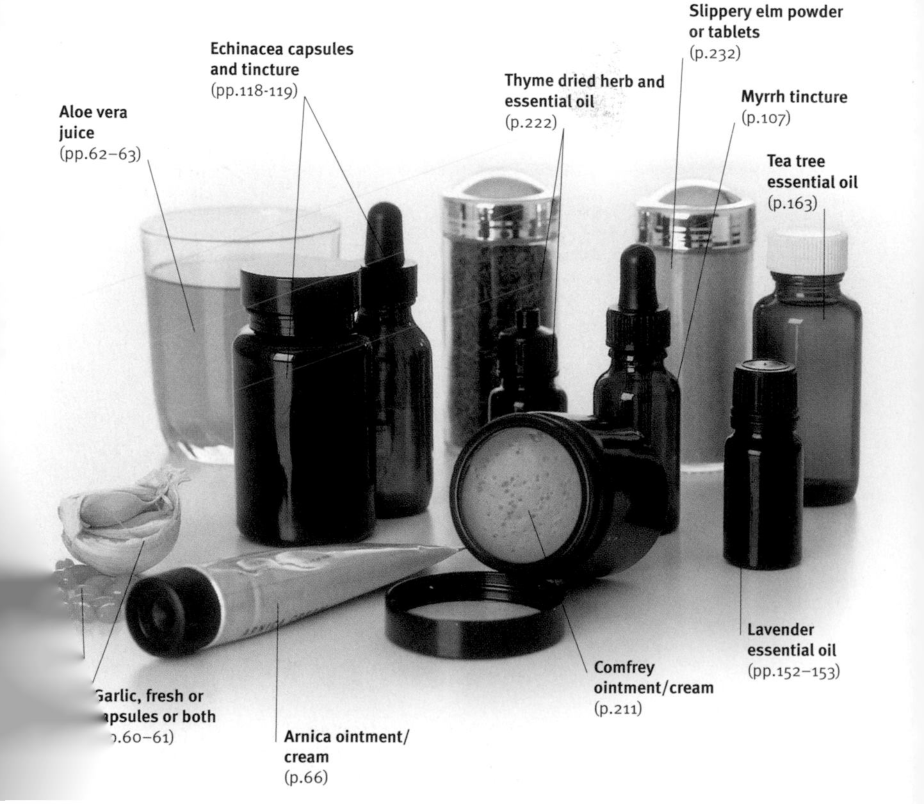

Slippery elm powder or tablets
(p.232)

Echinacea capsules and tincture
(pp.118-119)

Thyme dried herb and essential oil
(p.222)

Myrrh tincture
(p.107)

Aloe vera juice
(pp.62–63)

Tea tree essential oil
(p.163)

Lavender essential oil
(pp.152–153)

Garlic, fresh or capsules or both
(p.60–61)

Comfrey ointment/cream
(p.211)

Arnica ointment/ cream
(p.66)

Kitchen remedies

Not all remedies have to come out of a medicine bottle or jar. The kitchen shelf contains some of the best remedies for home treatment. Use cleaned, fresh produce, avoid old or discoloured material, and ensure storecupboard items are within their use-by date. Here are some examples:

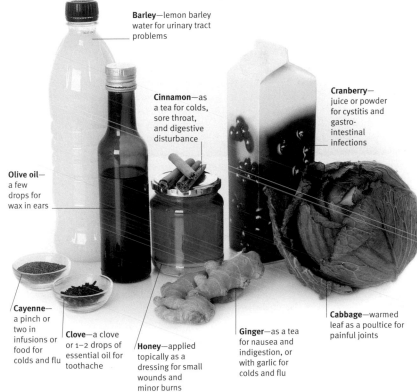

Barley—lemon barley water for urinary tract problems

Cinnamon—as a tea for colds, sore throat, and digestive disturbance

Cranberry—juice or powder for cystitis and gastro-intestinal infections

Olive oil—a few drops for wax in ears

Cayenne—a pinch or two in infusions or food for colds and flu

Clove—a clove or 1–2 drops of essential oil for toothache

Honey—applied topically as a dressing for small wounds and minor burns

Ginger—as a tea for nausea and indigestion, or with garlic for colds and flu

Cabbage—warmed leaf as a poultice for painful joints

HOME HERBAL PHARMACY

Any number of dried herbs or tinctures can be added to build up a home herbal pharmacy. The following are some of the more useful, versatile, and safe remedies:

Chamomile (*Chamomilla recutita*)
Cramp bark (*Viburnum opulus*)
Elderflower (*Sambucus nigra*)
Feverfew (*Tanacetum parthenium*)
Licorice (*Glycyrrhiza glabra*)
Lindenflower (*Tilia* spp.)
Meadowsweet (*Filipendula ulmaria*)
Peppermint (*Mentha x piperita*)
Rosemary (*Rosmarinus officinalis*)
Sage (*Salvia officinalis*)
Valerian (*Valeriana officinalis*)
Yarrow (*Achillea millefolium*)

THE HERB GARDEN

Growing herbs in the garden can bring real pleasure and a sense of achievement. Culinary herbs add zest to familiar recipes, and their scent lingers on summer evenings. At the same time, even a few medicinal herbs become a first aid resource for common health problems.

Outdoor pharmacy

Beyond the kitchen shelf and bathroom medicine cabinet, your home herbal pharmacy can extend out onto the window sill, balcony, or garden. Given adequate light, water, and food, many medicinal plants will thrive and a surprising number can be grown even in a small area. Living medicinal plants are a useful resource to have at hand; they are also a joy to work with and to have in the garden. Label plants so that when you are harvesting them you know precisely what material you are gathering.

If you are planting in the garden, choose herbs such as lemon balm (*Melissa officinalis*) or yarrow (*Achillea millefolium*) that grow vigorously in most soils and harvest well. Buying seeds or plants from specialist herb suppliers is usually the best way to stock a medicinal herb garden.

Other herbs that are readily cultivated at home include:
Calendula (*Calendula officinalis*)
Echinacea (*Echinacea* spp.)
Californian poppy (*Eschscholzia californica*)
Fennel (*Foeniculum vulgare*)
Lavender (*Lavandula* spp.)
Parsley (*Petroselinum crispum*)
Rosemary (*Rosmarinus officinalis*)
Sage (*Salvia officinalis*)
Thyme (*Thymus vulgaris*)
Feverfew (*Tanacetum parthenium*)
Vervain (*Verbena officinalis*)
Cranberry (*Vaccinium macrocarpon*).

CONTAINER HERBS

Many herbs will grow well in pots or other types of containers, including the following:

Lemon verbena (*Lippia citriodora*)
Peppermint (*Mentha x piperita*)
Oregano (*Origanum vulgare*)
Parsely (*Petroselinum crispum*)
Skullcap (*Scutellaria laoteriflora*)
Feverfew (*Tanacetum parthenium*)
Heartease (*Viola odorata*)
Basil (*Ocimum basilicum*)

THE RIGHT PLANT

Medicinal plant cultivation is fairly straightforward, but it is important to start with:
• The right plant species – *Aloe vera* is a safe and effective plant medicine, but some *Aloe* species are poisonous.
• The right variety – some varieties are more medicinally active than others. A specific variety of damiana (*Turnera diffusa* var. *aphrodisiaca*) is generally used.
• If the plant's essential oil is important, the right chemotype – plants of the same species and variety can differ in their chemical constituents, especially in their essential oils, for example lavender (*Lavandula angustifolia*).

HERB GARDEN
In a small plot, select herbs that have culinary and medicinal use such as fennel (*Foeniculum vulgare*), sage (*Salvia officinalis*), and thyme (*Thymus vulgaris*).

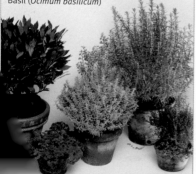

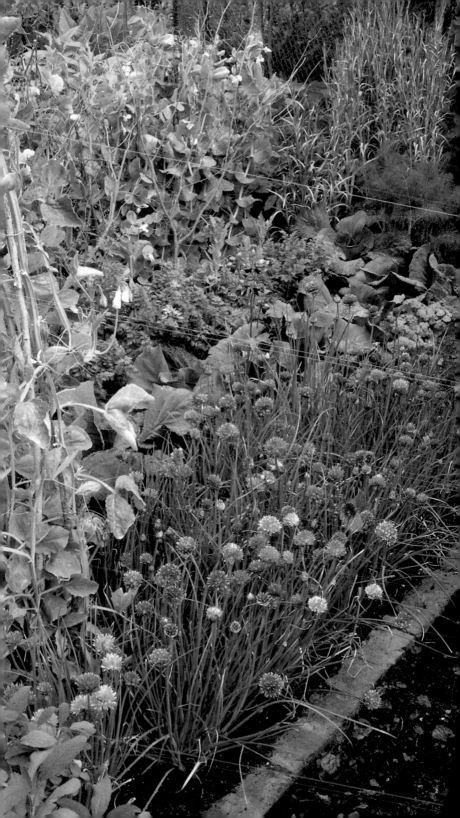

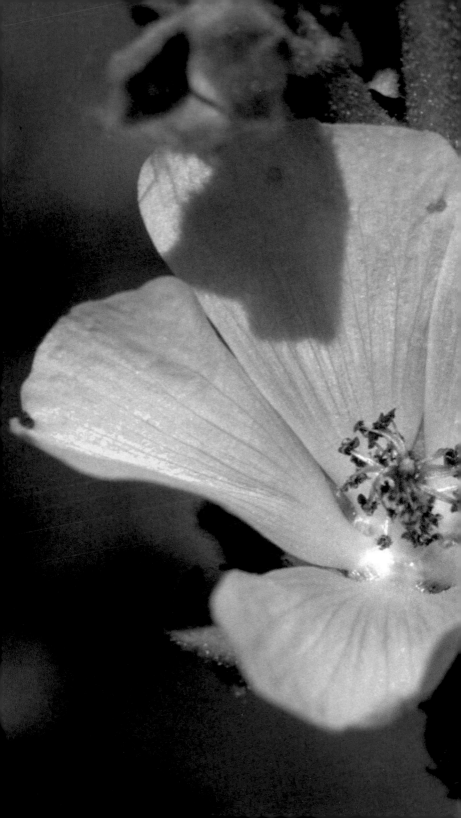

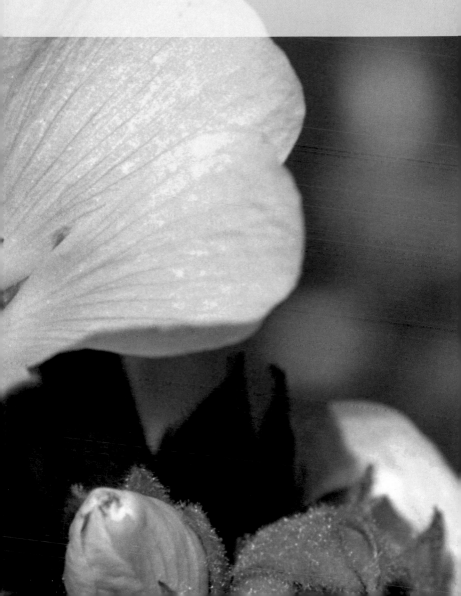

SAFETY AND QUALITY

SAFETY CONCERNS

Herbal remedies are natural but they are also medicines, and can cause side effects. Like all medicines, they need to be treated with respect and used carefully. The following section gives information and simple advice on the risks associated with taking herbal remedies.

SIDE EFFECTS

Herbal remedies have an excellent track record when it comes to safety, and side effects are very infrequent. However, unwanted reactions do occur and it is important to be alert to this possibility, especially when taking a remedy for the first time. Adverse reactions to herbal remedies usually involve minor symptoms such as digestive upset and headache. On stopping the remedy, symptoms usually clear slowly. Sometimes, existing symptoms can flare up when starting a new remedy.

In either case, if you suspect that you are reacting badly to an herbal remedy, stop taking it. If symptoms are severe, or continue to worsen despite stopping the remedy, seek immediate advice from your health care practitioner. If the symptoms are minor, try an alternative remedy.

Remedies that contain potentially irritant or toxic constituents, for example horse chestnut (*Aesculus hippocastanum*), are more likely to produce side effects and need to be treated with caution. Sticking to recommended dosage levels is important, especially in the case of children. Taking excessive doses of any medicine, whether herbal or conventional is likely to lead to side effects.

Allergic reactions to herbal medicines, even familiar ones such as German chamomile (*Chamomilla recutita*), are rare but do sometimes occur. Mild allergic reactions should begin to ease soon after contact with the remedy is ended—applying marigold (*Calendula officinalis*) cream and drinking nettle (*Urtica dioica*) tea can help with minor skin reactions. Severe allergic reactions are a medical emergency and need immediate medical attention.

For people who have allergies to plants or foods, or are known to be sensitive to medicines, it's a good policy to start new herbal remedies by taking a small amount, say half the minimum recommended dose. If everything is fine, build up over a few days to the standard dose; if it's not fine, stop!

Known cautions are listed for each herb in the A–Z of Herbal Remedies, pp.52–255.

HALF DOSE
If prone to allergies, start with a low dose.

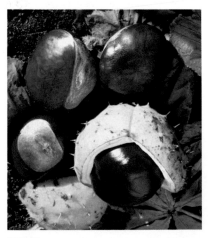

DOSAGE
Horse chestnut seed contains saponins that can irritate the gastrointenstinal tract. At the normal dosage, side effects are unlikely to occur.

CONTRAINDICATIONS

Some herbal remedies need to be avoided in preexisting health conditions, since they may worsen symptoms. For

LICORICE
The root contains constituents that stimulate the release of hormones by the adrenal glands. This action is mainly responsible for its effectiveness as an anti-inflammatory remedy.

example, people with high blood pressure should not take large doses of licorice (*Glycyrrhiza glabra*), because its action on the adrenal glands can lead to raised blood pressure. Licorice is therefore contraindicated in cases of high blood pressure—although, for the same reason, it may sometimes be a useful remedy in people with low blood pressure.

If you already have an existing unrelated health problem, remedies should be carefully selected in order to avoid using those that are contraindicated. Each remedy listed in the A–Z of Herbal Remedies can be checked for known contraindications.

Pregnancy and breast-feeding are the situations where herbal remedies are most commonly contraindicated. Some remedies are unsuitable to take during pregnancy and breast-feeding, and in the first three months of pregnancy all medication including herbal remedies should be avoided as far as possible. For more details, see Pregnancy and after on pp.46–47.

HERB–DRUG INTERACTIONS

Some herbs (and foods) influence the effects of conventional medicines, interacting with them and increasing or decreasing their strength of action. Often interaction between a herb, for

example schisandra (*Schisandra chinensis*) or cat's claw (*Uncaria tormentosa*) and a drug will be minor and go unnoticed, but in some cases herb-drug interactions can cause serious, even life-threatening problems.

The potential of St. John's wort (*Hypericum perforatum*) to interact with prescribed drugs has been intensively researched after it was found to speed up clearance of a number of drugs from the body. A report in *The Lancet* (2000) described the case of a heart transplant patient recovering well in the hospital who went quickly downhill after taking St. John's wort. On investigation it was discovered that St. John's wort had caused levels of ciclosporin, an immunosuppressant drug, to drop by 50 percent, leading his body to start rejecting his new heart. On ceasing to take St. John's wort, he quickly recovered.

This is an extreme example, but it illustrates that herb-drug interactions are real and need to be taken into account. If you are taking drugs prescribed by your doctor or hospital, check with them, or with a registered herbal or naturopathic practitioner, before taking an herbal remedy.

You can report an adverse reaction to a herbal remedy in the US at: http://www.fda.gov/medwatch/how.htm.

MAIN HERB–DRUG INTERACTIONS

The main categories of prescribed drugs requiring caution are:

- Anticoagulants, antidepressants, antiepileptics, and immunosuppressants; the effectiveness of oral contraceptives can also be affected.

- If you are taking prescribed medicines, do *not* stop taking them in order to start taking an herbal remedy. Seek professional advice from your doctor or herbal practitioner on the best way to proceed.

DOSAGE AND SENSIBLE USE

As with all medicines, getting the dosage right is essential. Too much and you risk overdosing, too little and the remedy may not work. Follow the guidelines on these pages to ensure that you use herbal remedies safely and appropriately.

ADULT DOSAGES

Each of the remedies listed in the A–Z of Herbal Remedies has a letter indicating its adult dosage—how much of the herb to take per day or per week.

To take an example, passion flower (*Passiflora incarnata*) on p.173 has C for its dosage. Looking at the dosage guide (*right*), it can be seen that C = 2–4g a day or 30g a week. Passion flower should therefore be taken at these recommended dosages.

As another example, hawthorn leaf (*Crataegus* spp.) has M and C for its dosage. M applies to manufactured products: take prepackaged hawthorn products, such as standardized tablets and capsules, at the manufacturer's recommended dosage. C applies to dried hawthorn leaf or berry: take at the recommended daily or weekly dosage, i.e. 2–4g a day or 30g a week.

Similarly, each of the other letters gives specific recommendations on how to use the herb.

Teas and decoctions The dosages given in the guide apply when making teas and decoctions from dried herb material—bark, leaves, roots, etc. For fresh herb material you can use 1½–2 times the quantity of dried material.

Tinctures It is not possible to give clear guidelines for tinctures owing to the wide variation in their strength. Ask advice on dosage when purchasing a tincture. In general, the dosage range for a 1:3 tincture is the same (in milliliters not grams) as the above dosages, i.e. for A, the dosage of a 1:3 tincture is 5–15ml a day

ADULT DOSAGE GUIDE

Recommended ADULT dosage as given in the key information boxes (*see opposite page*). For children and people over 70, see below and opposite.

A = 5–15g a day, or max. 100g (3½ oz) per week

B = 3–7.5g a day, or max. 50g (2 oz) per week

C = 2–4g a day, or max. 30g (1 oz) per week

D = 1–2g a day, or max. 15g (½ oz) per week

M = Take product at manufacturer's recommended dosage.

T = Topical application on the skin only (Note: preparations made specifically for topical use should not be taken internally.)

Powders Take the minimum recommended daily dosage only.

Tablets and capsules Take at the manufacturer's recommended dosage.

CHILDREN'S DOSAGES

Do not give babies under 6 months any medication without professional advice. You may need to adjust dosage levels for children who are particularly small or large for their age.

From 6 months to 1 year: give ⅒th the minimum adult dose
From 1 to 6 years: give ⅓rd the minimum adult dose
From 7 to 11 years: give ½ the minimum adult dose
From 12 to 16 years: give the low adult dose.

DOSAGES FOR OVER 70s

As we age, our bodies become less efficient at breaking down drugs, including herbs. From the age of about 70 onward it is advisable to take slightly lower doses: 80 percent of the standard adult dose is normally recommended. In very old and frail people the dosage may need to be as low as 50 percent of the standard adult dosage.

GENERAL CAUTIONS

- Do not take essential oils internally unless on advice of a suitably qualified health care professional.
- Do not give herbs to babies under 6 months old.
- Do not exceed the recommended dosage levels.

- If you are taking drugs prescribed by your doctor or hospital, check with them, or with a registered herbal or naturopathic practitioner, before taking a herbal remedy.
- People known to have allergies should start by taking a low dose and, if this is fine, then increase the dose.
- Contact allergy can occur on handling fresh or dried herbs. Where such allergy occurs, do not take the remedy internally. Some people are allergic to specific plant families, for example the daisy (*Asteraceae*) family. Several herbs listed in this book, including chamomile (*Chamomilla recutita*), echinacea (*Echinacea* spp.), and feverfew (*Tanacetum parthenium*), belong to this family and are known to cause contact allergy in sensitive individuals.

Key information

Every remedy in the A–Z features a key information box that provides essential data on the herb. At the top, each herb is rated using a 5 star-rating system, with 5 black stars = most. This gives some idea of the herb's:
- overall safety record (Safety)
- long-standing use in traditional medicine (Traditional use)
- evidence of effectiveness, as supported by scientific research (Research).

On the line below (Best taken as), suitable types of preparation are recommended; for example, yarrow (*Achillea millefolium*) is best taken as a tea, which gets 3 checks. Dosage information is provided on the following line. Some entries include an "Often used with" recommendation. The last and most important section lists known cautions for the remedy, and should be read carefully, especially before taking a remedy.

	KEY INFORMATION
overall level of safety	**SAFETY** ★★★★☆
use of herb supported by research	**TRADITIONAL USE** ★★★★★ — use in herbal medicine
	RESEARCH ★★★★★
	BEST TAKEN AS Fresh raw garlic ✓✓✓ — the best form to take the herb
	Whole garlic extract/aged garlic (as tablet or capsule) ✓✓
guidelines on dosage	**DOSAGE** Long-term: 1 clove a day; short-term: up to 3 cloves a day; manufactured products: M (*see pp.44–45*)
common herbal combinations	**OFTEN USED WITH** Echinacea species (*Echinacea*)
	CAUTIONS If taking anticoagulants (blood-thinning drugs) such as aspirin or warfarin, take garlic only on the advice of a herbal or medical practitioner. See also pp.42–51. — safety guidelines

PREGNANCY AND AFTER

Herbal medicine has an important role to play as part of a natural approach to health care for expectant mothers and their children. While caution is required in avoiding potentially harmful remedies, many gentle-acting herbs can safely be used during pregnancy and beyond.

Herbal medicines pre- and postnatally

Herbal remedies can be safe to take during pregnancy, although for the first three months of pregnancy, they should be taken only after consulting a professional. From the fourth month onward, a range of safe and effective remedies may be used to treat simple health problems such as colds and constipation. Select remedies with a long history of use in pregnancy and with no evidence of risk to mother or baby. The box below gives examples.

Check labels of herbal products carefully, especially where herbs and other constituents are combined together. Alcohol should be avoided during the first three months, even in the small amounts present in tinctures. It is much better to use teas, decoctions, tablets, or capsules.

HERBS TO AVOID

Some of the herbs included in this book are contraindicated and unsafe to take during pregnancy and while breast-feeding. In particular, do not take:
• Chiretta (*Andrographis paniculata*)
• Neem (*Azadirachta indica*)
• Goldenseal (*Hydrastis canadensis*)
• Lobelia (*Lobelia inflata*)
• Butterbur (*Petasites hybridus*)
• Pau d'arco (*Tabebuia impetiginosa*)
• Coltsfoot (*Tussilago farafara*).

Essential oils, and herbs that contain strong essential oils such as eucalyptus (*Eucalyptus* spp.), thuja (*Thuja occidentalis*), and sage (*Salvia officinalis*), are also contraindicated and should not be used during pregnancy and while breast-feeding.

SOME HERBS COMMONLY USED IN PREGNANCY AND WHILE BREAST-FEEDING

When pregnant and while breast-feeding, check the relevant cautions before taking a remedy. Remember that herbs are passed on to the baby in breast milk.

Garlic (*Allium sativum*)
Calendula (*Calendula officinalis*)
Senna (*Cassia* spp.)
Chamomile (*Chamomilla recutita*)
Echinacea (*Echinacea* spp.)
* Raspberry leaf (*Rubus ideaus*)
Butcher's broom (*Ruscus aculeatus*)
Elderflower/berry (*Sambucus nigra*)
Limeflowers (*Tilia* spp.)
Nettle (*Urtica dioica*)
Slippery elm (*Ulmus fulva*)
Bilberry (*Vaccinium myrtillus*)
Cramp bark (*Viburnum opulus*)
Ginger (*Zingiber officinalis*)
Cornsilk (*Zea mays*)

* Take raspberry leaf only in the last 3 months of pregnancy; see also pp.191.

Herbal medicines and children

By and large children respond very well to herbal remedies, even if the taste can make administering them a bit of a struggle! Adding honey or mixing with apple juice will usually help make remedies more palatable. Tablets or capsules can usually be opened and ground up, and taken on a spoon mixed with honey, maple syrup, and so forth.

Children typically fall ill and recover quickly. This can be very alarming for parents, since a healthy child at 8:00 am can be a very unwell one by 11:00 am. The main worry in acute illness is controlling fever and keeping the temperature below 102°F (39°C). Children with fevers approaching this level (and above) need medical attention.

That being said, the very unwell child at 2:00 pm can be running around again by 6:00 pm; children bounce back. Get to know your child's typical pattern when falling ill—you will often be able to recognize the difference between day-to-day problems and a potentially serious illness. The former can be safely treated with herbal remedies, while the latter needs professional advice and treatment. If in doubt, always err on the side of caution and seek advice.

SOME HERBAL REMEDIES SUITABLE FOR CHILDREN

Guidelines on dosage levels for children are given in Dosage and sensible use, pp.44–45.

Garlic (*Allium sativum*)
Marshmallow (*Althea officinalis*)
Caraway (*Carum carvi*)
Chamomile (*Chamomilla recutita*)
Echinacea (*Echinacea* spp.)
Californian poppy (*Eschscholzia californica*)
Cinnamon (*Cinnamonum verum*)
Eyebright (*Euphrasia officinalis*)
Meadowsweet (*Filipendula ulmaria*)
Sea buckthorn (*Hippophae rhamnoides*)
Elecampane (*Inula helenium*)
Plantain (*Plantago* spp.)
Blackcurrant (*Ribes nigra*)
Yellow dock (*Rumex crispus*)
Elderflower/berry (*Sambucus nigra*)
Thyme (*Thymus vulgaris*)
Linden flowers (*Tilia* spp.)
Red clover (*Trifolium pratense*)
Slippery elm (*Ulmus fulva*)
Nettle (*Urtica dioica*)

BABIES UP TO 6 MONTHS
Herbs are not safe for young babies, but breast-feeding mothers can take suitable remedies for them.

TIPS FOR HOME USE

Self-treatment of minor health problems makes sense, and besides helping one to feel better, can be very satisfying. These pages give a few tips on how to refine the use of herbal remedies. In cases of more serious illness, it is wise to consult a qualified herbal practitioner.

How to choose the right remedy

- Decide what the main symptoms are.
- Select remedies that are known to help these symptoms, for example cranberry (*Vaccinium macrocarpon*) for cystitis, elderflower (*Sambucus nigra*) for colds and sinus congestion.
- Develop experience using specific remedies and build up your own stock of herbal remedies.

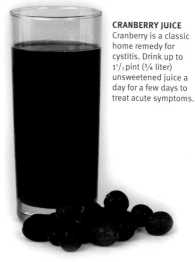

CRANBERRY JUICE
Cranberry is a classic home remedy for cystitis. Drink up to 1$^1/_3$ pint (¾ liter) unsweetened juice a day for a few days to treat acute symptoms.

HOW MANY TO USE

- Combining 2–4 herbal remedies together can prove more effective, particularly if the problem is stubborn or recurs frequently; for example recurrent cystitis infection may be treated with cranberry, plus remedies such as buchu (*Barosma betulina*), echinacea (*Echinacea* spp.), and cornsilk (*Zea mays*).
- Combine remedies as teas or tinctures, or purchase a product containing the required remedies.

WHEN AND HOW MUCH TO TAKE

- Herbal remedies are generally best taken with water about 30 minutes before a meal.
- Take the recommended daily amount in 2–3 divided doses, ideally before your breakfast, lunch, and evening meal.
- Moderate to high doses of an herb can be taken for a few days for minor acute problems, for example if you are experiencing a sudden onset of cystitis symptoms, take cornsilk at the upper end of its dosage range (10–15g a day) for 3–4 days.
- Low to moderate doses should be used for long-term problems, for example in the case of chronic bladder irritation, take cornsilk regularly at a low dosage (5–7.5g a day).

HOW LONG TO TAKE FOR

- Self-limiting conditions such as a sore throat or stomach upset that are safe to treat at home should clear within 10–14 days at the most. If you are not fully recovered by then, see your health care practitioner.
- Start treatment as soon as possible, before symptoms become full-blown.
- Some remedies may be taken long-term to prevent or treat chronic illness, for example ginkgo (*Ginkgo biloba*) to maintain healthy mental function or boswellia (*Boswellia serrata*) to provide relief for arthritic pain and stiffness.

When to seek professional advice

- Do not put off getting professional advice when symptoms are worrying, especially if severe pain or a temperature of over 102°F (39°C) are present, or if symptoms deteriorate sharply or unexpectedly. Professional advice, including telephone help lines, will help ensure that you have the right treatment at the right time.
- More detailed guidance on when to seek professional advice is given in Common Health Problems, pp.256–275.

HOW CAN AN HERBAL PRACTITIONER HELP?

- Herbal practitioners are trained, often at university, to use their in-depth knowledge of herbal medicine to assess and treat a wide range of health problems. They are able to give detailed advice on the best remedies and products to use, together with appropriate advice on diet and lifestyle. Where appropriate, they will refer to other practitioners, including medical doctors, and can advise on interactions between herbs and drugs.
- If you have ongoing health problems, or want access to natural health care

WHAT HEALTH PROBLEMS DO HERBALISTS TREAT BEST?

Herbal practitioners specialize in treating health problems with herbal medicine, and give advice on diet and supplements. The following types of conditions often benefit from treatment:

- allergies
- anxiety and stress-related problems
- arthritic and rheumatic conditions
- chronic infection and fatigue
- chronic inflammatory diseases
- mild to moderate depression
- digestive complaints
- menstrual and menopausal problems
- skin disorders

for your family, contact herbal practitioners in your area and find one with whom you feel comfortable and you trust. Check that your practitioner, or medical herbalist, is insured and a member of a professional body such as the American Herbalists Guild in the US. He or she should provide you with details of likely costs of initial and follow-up consultations and herbs.

HERBAL DISPENSARY
Medical herbalists stock a wide range of medicines. Each patient receives an individually tailored prescription, normally dispensed on the spot.

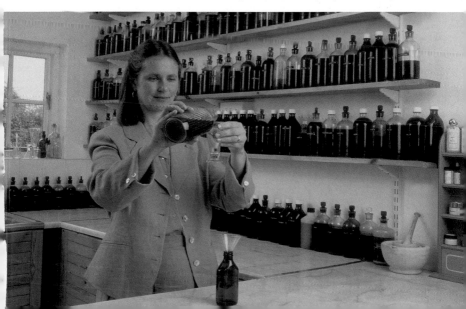

HOW TO BUY REMEDIES

When buying a remedy, select a suitable herb or combination for your health problem, such as feverfew (*Tanacetum parthenium*) for migraine headaches. Decide how you want to take it, for example as a capsule, and compare the different products available.

Where to obtain herbal remedies

Most people working with herbal medicine recommend buying remedies from a reputable health food shop or pharmacy. Try to find a shop that specializes in natural medicines, where the staff is knowledgeable and receives regular in-house training. Their advice can help to guide you toward buying appropriate, good-quality remedies. Shops that sell dried herbs and dispense tinctures are likely to have the most knowledgeable staff and should be actively concerned to supply good-quality herbal produce. Do not be afraid to ask how they can be sure that the products they sell are of good quality.

Buying remedies from an herbal practitioner is also a reliable way of obtaining them. He or she will stock products from growers and suppliers with a long-established record of quality control. Remember that the ethical code of a professional herbalist prevents him or her from selling you an herbal remedy without a consultation, for which you will usually have to pay. This is to check up on your health and make sure that you receive the right advice for your situation. However, you will probably find that herbs supplied by a practitioner compare favorably in cost and quality with herbs obtained elsewhere.

Herbal remedies can also be purchased via mail order or the Internet, and in some cases you can source innovative products that are hard to find in a local health food shop. However, it can be very hard to distinguish between suppliers of genuine products and those that are there for the quick sale. Some mail order and Internet companies deliberately base themselves in countries where proper quality control can be bypassed.

Where they are available, choosing organically certified herbal medicines makes sense on several counts, as plants are grown free of pesticides and pollutants, sites are regularly inspected, and the harvesting of organic herbs supports conservation in the wild.

QUALITY AND VALUE FOR MONEY

The price of herbal remedies is directly linked to quality. As a general rule, buy remedies produced by specialist herbal companies or well-known manufacturers, where effective quality control should be routine. Retailers who consistently market remedies at prices lower than the norm are either taking a loss or selling products of doubtful quality! The best-value remedies are often sold at middle-of-the-road prices, reflecting acceptable quality. In some cases, for example ginseng (*Panax ginseng*), genuine high-quality products are available, and the higher price reflects this.

Sadly, poor-quality herbal products are still commonplace. If you take St. John's wort (*Hypericum perforatum*) for mild to moderate depression, for example, it is reasonable to expect some signs of improvement. If no change occurs, this might be due to poor quality. Try a different product, perhaps a tea or tincture, instead.

BUYING DRIED HERBS

If you are purchasing dried plant material, bear in mind that herbs will soon deteriorate if they are not stored properly:

- Herbs should be stored in clear glass jars or brown paper bags, kept out of direct sunlight and away from damp or heat.
- Good-quality herbs should have their distinctive smell and taste—

for example, marigold should be a vibrant orange color, nettle leaf a deep dark green.

- Old or poorly dried herbs will be faded and will have lost their normal color.
- Do not buy dried herbs in greater quantity than you need.

For the pros and cons of different herbal preparations, see Types of herbal remedy on pp. 30–33.

What the label should tell you

Different countries have different regulations governing what can (or cannot) be put on product labels. Nevertheless, any herbal product worth buying should have the information shown in the example below printed on the label or included as an insert.

In general, you should select herbal remedies that provide all this information; avoid buying products on which it is lacking. In particular, do not buy products where neither the local nor the botanical names of the herbs are given.

CHECKING THE LABEL
A reputable herbal product should give all the information shown in this example. When looking at similar products, compare the amount of herb material each provides. Also check to see what part of the plant has been used.

the names of all herbs and other constituents in the product

safety issues

recommended minimum and maximum dosage

contact details of manufacturer or supplier

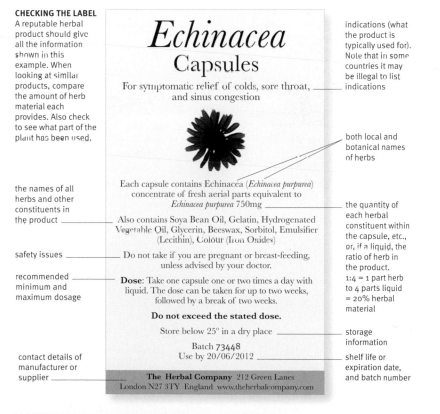

Echinacea
Capsules
For symptomatic relief of colds, sore throat, and sinus congestion

Each capsule contains Echinacea (*Echinacea purpurea*) concentrate of fresh aerial parts equivalent to
Echinacea purpurea 750mg

Also contains Soya Bean Oil, Gelatin, Hydrogenated Vegetable Oil, Glycerin, Beeswax, Sorbitol, Emulsifier (Lecithin), Colour (Iron Oxides)

Do not take if you are pregnant or breast-feeding, unless advised by your doctor.

Dose: Take one capsule one or two times a day with liquid. The dose can be taken for up to two weeks, followed by a break of two weeks.

Do not exceed the stated dose.

Store below 25° in a dry place

Batch 73448
Use by 20/06/2012

The Herbal Company 212 Green Lanes
London N27 3TY England www.theherbalcompany.com

indications (what the product is typically used for). Note that in some countries it may be illegal to list indications

both local and botanical names of herbs

the quantity of each herbal constituent within the capsule, etc., or, if a liquid, the ratio of herb in the product.
1:4 = 1 part herb to 4 parts liquid = 20% herbal material

storage information

shelf life or expiration date, and batch number

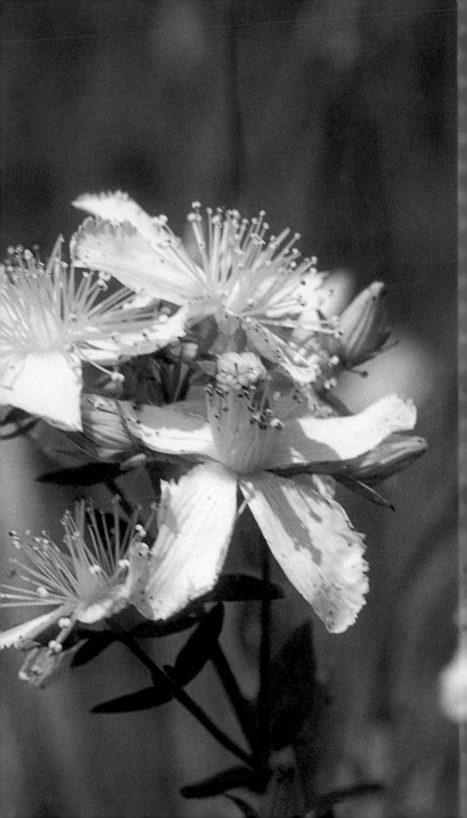

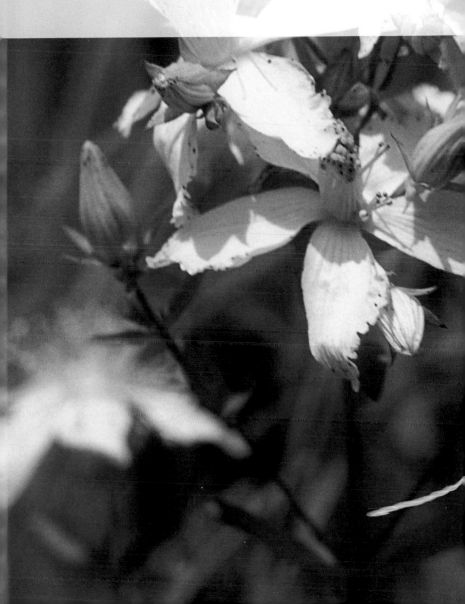

A-Z OF HERBAL REMEDIES

Yarrow

Achillea millefolium

Used as something of a cure-all, yarrow is an excellent remedy for colds, flu, and fever. It is equally good for healing cuts and bruises and slowing or stopping bleeding, for example, nosebleed. The Ancient Greek hero Achilles reputedly used yarrow on his wounded troops during the Trojan War.

MEDICINAL USES

Parts used Aerial parts ● Leaf

Key actions Astringent ● Digestive tonic ● Stimulates sweating and reduces fever ● Stops bleeding ● Strengthens blood vessels (especially veins) ● Wound healer

Colds, flu, and fever Yarrow is most commonly taken as a tea to ease cold and flu symptoms, control associated fever, and speed recovery. Drink the tea hot, since this strongly stimulates sweating and encourages cooling. Increased sweating can help to reduce fever and leads to improved cleansing of waste products from the body. It combines particularly well with elderflower (*Sambucus nigra*).

In the Scottish Highlands, Yarrow was traditionally made into an ointment and applied as a salve to heal wounds and bruises, and treat skin problems.

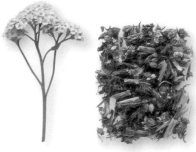

FLOWERS   DRIED AERIAL PARTS

aerial parts are used to relieve colds and flu

Other uses As a mild bitter, yarrow stimulates appetite and digestive activity, and is useful in treating diarrhea and irritable bowel syndrome. It will help to reduce heavy menstrual bleeding and aids menstrual regularity. Yarrow is also a remedy for the circulation, helping to lower blood pressure, strengthen capillaries (small blood vessels), and tone varicose veins. Topically, the tea can be applied as a lotion to small cuts and abrasions.

KEY INFORMATION

SAFETY   ★ ★ ★ ☆ ☆
TRADITIONAL USE   ★ ★ ★ ★ ★
RESEARCH   ★ ☆ ☆ ☆ ☆
    BEST TAKEN AS Tea ✓✓✓
    Tincture ✓✓ Capsule ✓
    DOSAGE B (*see pp.44–45*)
    OFTEN USED WITH Elderflower
    (*Sambucus nigra*).
CAUTIONS Allergic reactions can occur (especially skin irritation); not advisable during pregnancy and while breast-feeding; not advisable for children under 5. See also pp.42–51.

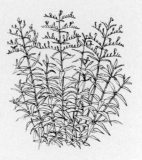

Chiretta

Andrographis paniculata

Native to India, chiretta has a powerfully bitter taste that stimulates digestive and liver activity and counters infection. Highly valued in both Ayurvedic and Chinese medicine, its traditional uses include serious health problems such as dysentery, fever, leprosy, malaria, and worms.

MEDICINAL USES

Part used Whole plant

Key actions Anti-inflammatory
● Bitter tonic ● Immune-stimulant
● Protects liver

Poor immune system, liver and digestive problems An herb that has been becoming increasingly well-known in the West, chiretta has a therapeutic profile that is almost unique. On the one hand, it supports and strengthens the liver, protecting it from infection and toxic damage, while on the other, it has a marked ability to stimulate the body's immune system, making it more able to ward off and resist infection, especially viral infection. While the herb has mostly been used for liver problems in the past, its immune-enhancing properties make it a key remedy for protecting against upper respiratory infections, including colds, flu-like colds, and influenza.

Several good-quality clinical trials have concluded that chiretta can reduce symptoms and improve the rate of recovery in people suffering from sinusitis, flu-like colds, and throat infection. It can also be helpful in gastrointestinal problems, such as food poisoning, gastroenteritis, and diarrhea. Studies suggest that chiretta is as effective as paracetamol in relieving flu and fever symptoms, taken consistently over several days for best results. Chiretta is best taken on professional advice in liver disorders, and it works well with other liver remedies, such as milk thistle (*Silybum marianum*). Chiretta is also being investigated for its ability to help prevent cancer.

KEY INFORMATION

SAFETY ★ ★ ★ ★ ☆
TRADITIONAL USE ★ ★ ★ ★ ☆
RESEARCH ★ ★ ★ ☆ ☆
BEST TAKEN AS Tablet ✓✓✓ Capsule ✓✓
Tincture ✓
DOSAGE B: infusion, tincture.
Andrographis extract (standardized to 4% andrographolides) as tablets: 1020mg a day (*see pp.44–45*)
OFTEN USED WITH Echinacea (*Echinacea* spp.)
CAUTIONS Excess dosage may cause digestive discomfort; do not take during pregnancy and while breast-feeding. See also pp.42–51.

CAPSULES

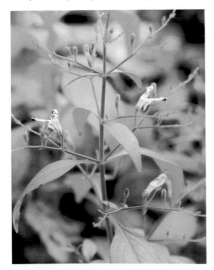

While chiretta is used principally as an immune-enhancing remedy in the West, it is seen mainly as a digestive remedy in Ayurvedic and Chinese medicine.

Horse chestnut

Aesculus hippocastanum

Originally from southeastern Europe and Asia, the horse chestnut or "conker" tree is known around much of the world, although its health benefits are less well recognized. The shiny brown seeds—poisonous if eaten—are processed to make an effective medicine for the veins.

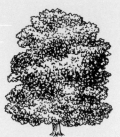

MEDICINAL USES

Part used Seed

Key actions Anti-inflammatory
● Astringent ● Reduces fluid retention
● Vein tonic

Venous circulatory problems

Horse chestnut is a major remedy for the veins and capillaries. As an astringent and anti-inflammatory, it has a beneficial effect on veins throughout the body, tightening up and toning the vein walls where they have become damaged and sore. By drawing back fluid that has leaked out of veins, horse chestnut reduces swelling and congestion in veins, as well as local inflammation, and is the first choice in herbal treatment for

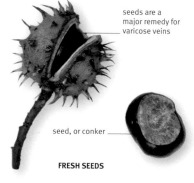

seeds are a
major remedy for
varicose veins

seed, or conker

FRESH SEEDS

varicose veins and venous insufficiency (poor vein health). It is usually taken as a standardized tablet or capsule, although it may also be applied to the skin overlying varicose veins as a lotion, ointment, or gel. It should not be applied on broken or ulcerated skin. Its effectiveness has been fairly well established, though it usually needs to be

The horse chestnut is found worldwide in temperate regions, and is widely grown in northern and western Europe as an ornamental tree.

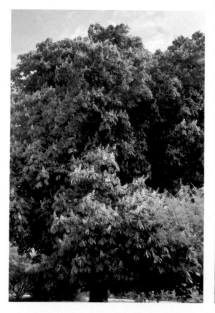

HORSE SENSE

In Turkey, horse chestnut was used to treat chest problems in horses, donkeys, and mules, and its common name may derive from this practice. As early as the 16th century, herbalists noted that "Turks call them horse chestnuts because they are very helpful for treating panting horses."

taken for several months for signs of improvement, as healing venous circulation can be a very difficult task. A clinical trial at London's Barts Hospital in 1996 showed that horse chestnut extract was as effective as a compression stocking in treating varicose veins in the leg.

Other uses Horse chestnut may be used to treat other problems affecting the veins, for example, hemorrhoids and thread veins, and can be useful in treating leg cramps, and swelling and fluid retention in the legs. It may be taken to treat conditions such as deep vein thrombosis, frostbite, and leg ulcers, but only on professional advice. As a preventative, it will help reduce the risks of deep vein thrombosis, for example on long flights. An oil extracted from the conkers has been used as a topical application for rheumatism in France, while in the US, a decoction of the leaves has been considered useful for pertussis.

leaves may be used as a cough remedy

Although seeds are the most commonly used plant part, a decoction of the bark can be used in place of the seed as an astringent lotion for varicose veins.

KEY INFORMATION

SAFETY	★ ★ ★ ☆ ☆
TRADITIONAL USE	★ ★ ★ ★ ☆
RESEARCH	★ ★ ★ ★ ☆

BEST TAKEN AS Standardized extract (tablet) ✓✓✓

DOSAGE Tincture: C (*see pp.44–45*) Tablet: 90–150mg of standardized extract (16–21% triterpene glycosides [aescin] a day)

OFTEN USED WITH Butcher's broom (*Ruscus aculeatus*)

CAUTIONS Not suitable for children; may cause digestive irritation (not in enteric-coated preparations). If pregnant or breast-feeding, or taking blood-thinning medication, consult an herbal or medical practitioner. See also pp.42–51.

Cultivated as an ornamental tree in temperate regions of the world, the horse chestnut (*Aesculus hippocastanum*), has spiny green fruit with brown seeds, which are used medicinally.

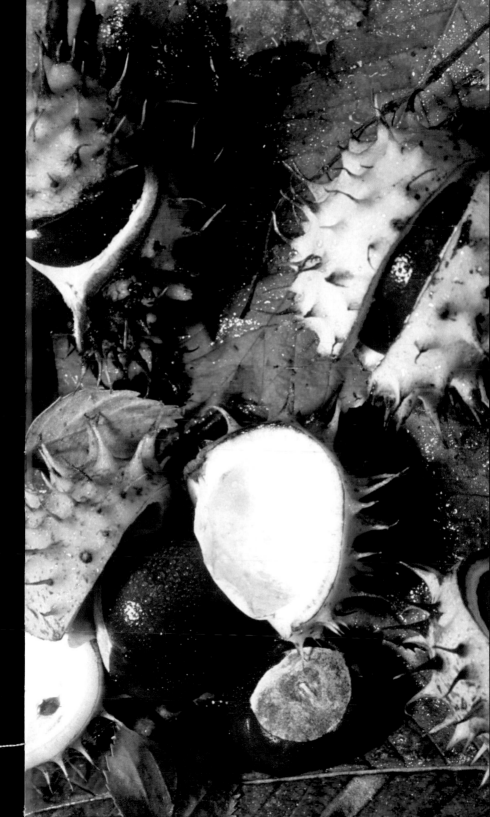

Garlic

Allium sativum

One of the world's most important medicinal plants, garlic is also one of the most researched, with over 1,000 published papers investigating its therapeutic activity. Folklore has it that garlic protects against the devil and vampires, beliefs that attest to its power as a medicine, particularly in countering infection.

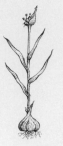

MEDICINAL USES

Part used Clove (one segment of the bulb)

Key actions Antibiotic • Antifungal • Blood-thinner • Counters cough and respiratory infection • Lowers blood pressure • Lowers cholesterol levels • Supports beneficial intestinal flora

Infections Before modern antibiotics became commonly available, garlic was one of the most frequently used remedies to treat infection. In World War I, it was used to dress battle wounds. Although we have far more potent antibiotics today, garlic still has a place in treating infection. It makes an excellent remedy for all types of respiratory infections, including sinusitis, cold, flu, sore throat, cough,

a tonic food
and medicine

has antiseptic
volatile oil

BULB   **CLOVE**

increase resistance
to infection

GARLIC PEARLS

and, more specifically, bronchitis. Swallowed whole (one small clove), eaten crushed in with food, or taken as a tablet, garlic will strengthen the body's ability to fight infection and speed recovery. A simple and effective kitchen remedy for colds, sore throats, and coughs can be readily made by mixing a crushed clove of garlic with freshly squeezed lemon juice (*Citrus limon*), 1–2 teaspoons of honey, and a pinch of dried ginger (*Zingiber officinalis*) powder or, preferably, a small piece of chopped fresh ginger root. Place in a mug, add hot water, and stir. Drink up to three cups a day. Garlic may be taken alongside, and is likely to complement prescribed antibiotics, at the same time warding off possible side effects by helping to protect beneficial intestinal bacteria and reducing the chances of developing thrush. Applied consistently over several weeks, fresh garlic or garlic oil may prove successful in countering

KEY INFORMATION

SAFETY	★ ★ ★ ★ ☆
TRADITIONAL USE	★ ★ ★ ★ ★
RESEARCH	★ ★ ★ ★ ★

BEST TAKEN AS Fresh raw garlic ✓✓✓ Whole garlic extract/aged garlic (as tablet or capsule) ✓✓
DOSAGE Long-term: 1 clove a day; short-term: up to 3 cloves a day; manufactured products: M (*see pp.44–45*)
OFTEN USED WITH Echinacea species (*Echinacea*)
CAUTIONS If taking anti-coagulants (blood-thinning drugs) such as aspirin, take garlic only on the advice of an herbal or medical practitioner. See also pp.42–51.

local fungal infections, such as itchy ear passages and warts.

Circulatory problems Despite its varied uses, garlic is today most valued for its positive effects on the circulation. Taken long-term, garlic helps to prevent atherosclerosis (furring up and narrowing of the arteries), thins the blood, and supports better cholesterol levels. These effects promote a more efficient circulation through the

CHOPPED CLOVES

A bulbous perennial originally from central Asia, garlic is now cultivated commercially worldwide for its use in cooking.

> ### GARLIC OIL
>
> To make garlic oil, crush or finely chop 4 large cloves and place them in a small non-stick pan. Add 3 tablespoons of organic olive oil. Heat gently until the mixture is just simmering then simmer for 1–2 minutes, stirring constantly. Pour the contents into a glass jar and leave to cool. Strain, bottle, and label. Use within 12 months.

arteries, support a lower blood pressure, and reduce the risk of heart problems.

Cancer When taken long-term, garlic also has a firm reputation as a preventative against cancer.

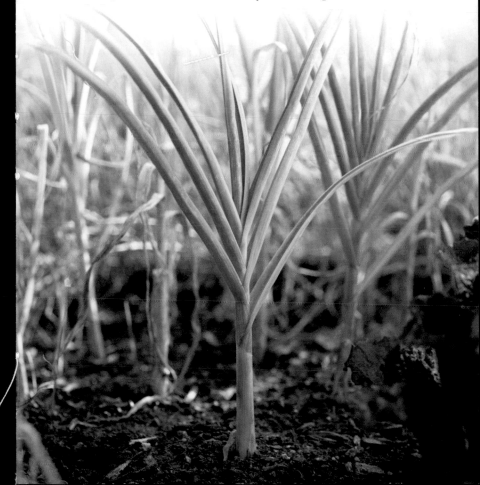

Aloe vera

Aloe vera

Grown throughout the tropics—and on window sills in cold areas—the thick, spiky, and fleshy leaves of aloe vera yield a cooling gel that makes an excellent treatment for minor burns and abrasions. Known in the United States as a "first aid plant," it should be grown in every kitchen as a handy first aid remedy.

MEDICINAL USES

Part used Leaf

Key actions Anti-inflammatory
• Immune support • Skin toner
• Wound and tissue healer

Skin conditions, wounds, and burns

Aloe vera has been prized as a medicine for several thousand years, and is now one of the most commonly used of all herbal remedies. Aloe vera's combination of potent healing and anti-inflammatory activity make it ideal for stimulating repair of damaged tissue, whether resulting from trauma—for example, burns or bruising from a blow—or otherwise. The gel or lotion can be applied neat to sore and inflamed skin, and may be used topically in a wide range of conditions, including acne, dermatitis, herpes sores, nappy rash, nettle rash, psoriasis, radiation burn (after radiotherapy, for example), shingles, and sunburn. For minor burns, first run the affected area under cold tap water for at least 10 minutes, then bathe in aloe vera gel. As a rule, aloe vera is best not applied to open wounds. Like the other powerful herbal wound healer comfrey (*Symphytum officinale*), aloe vera has a

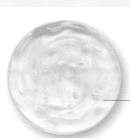

gel is a first aid remedy for burns

ALOE VERA GEL

reputation for promoting effective wound healing that minimizes the likelihood of scar (keloid) formation. It combines well with comfrey in healing deep-seated problems such as fractures and sports injuries.

Mouth and throat problems Aloe vera makes an effective wash for all manner of problems occurring within the mouth. Dab the gel onto mouth ulcers or aching teeth. Rinse the mouth and gums daily with gel to help heal gingivitis and to tone receding gums. Aloe vera gel, combined perhaps with sage (*Salvia officinalis*) tea, will make a

KEY INFORMATION

SAFETY	★★★★✩
TRADITIONAL USE	★★★★★
RESEARCH	★★★★☆

BEST TAKEN AS Fresh gel or lotion (topically), prepared juice (internally) ✓✓✓
DOSAGE Aloe vera concentrate: M (*see pp.44–45*)
CAUTIONS The gel can cause an allergic reaction; when using for the first time, apply a small quantity to the skin to test the response. Take internally only after consulting an herbal or medical practitioner. See also pp.42–51.

contains healing clear gel

LEAF

Grow aloe vera in a warm location, water sparingly, and you will have an excellent first aid remedy at hand whenever needed. To release the gel, cut the leaf with a sharp knife about 3in (7.5cm) from the tip. On a worksurface, carefully slice up the middle of the leaf. Peel back the two sides and expose the clear gel inside. Collect the clear gel and apply as required. Do not use the yellow sap released at the side of the leaf.

FRESH LEAF

Aloe vera thrives in a warm site with indirect sunlight. Like all succulents, it hates being overwatered; allow the soil to dry out in between waterings.

useful gargle for sore throat and hoarseness, especially where recovery is proving slow.

Other uses A different part of the leaf yields a latex and, taken internally, it has longstanding traditional use in treating stomach and duodenal ulcers and irritable bowel syndrome. A growing body of research indicates that aloe vera has a positive stimulant effect on the immune system, with clinical trials suggesting possible benefits in conditions as varied as asthma and HIV. Many species of aloe vera are used in medicine; some of them are potentially toxic. Quality control is very important when considering taking aloe vera gel internally. For this reason, it is recommended to take aloe vera internally on professional advice only.

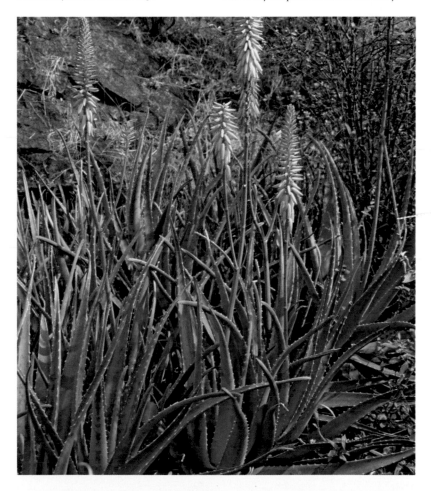

With a long history of use in skin treatments—Cleopatra attributed her beauty to it—aloe vera (*Aloe vera*) is today grown worldwide for the healing clear gel from its leaves.

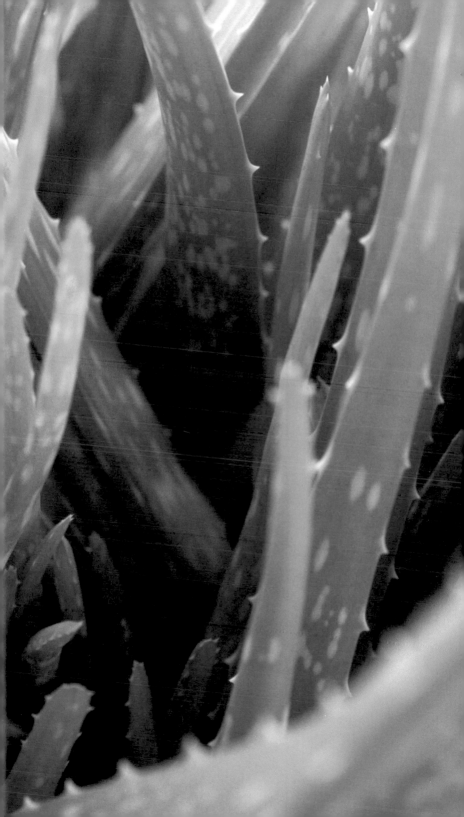

Marshmallow

Althea officinalis

A traditional European herb, marshmallow has soothing and calming properties that are mostly used to treat digestive and respiratory disorders.

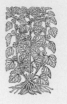

MEDICINAL USES

Parts used Flower ● Leaf ● Root

Key actions Demulcent and emollient ● Expectorant

Inflamed mucous membranes
Marshmallow root is typically used to soothe and protect irritated mucous membranes in, for example, acid indigestion, irritable bowel syndrome, and chronic bronchitis. Its sticky consistency means that it works like the body's own mucus to reduce discomfort and inflammation.

FLOWER

Other uses The leaf is preferred for urinary tract problems such as mild cystitis. The flower soothes the skin and contains high levels of antioxidants.

KEY INFORMATION

SAFETY	★ ★ ★ ★ ★
TRADITIONAL USE	★ ★ ★ ★ ☆
RESEARCH	★ ★ ★ ☆ ☆

BEST TAKEN AS Infusion, decoction ✓✓✓
DOSAGE A (*see pp.44–45*)
CAUTIONS None known. See also pp.42–51.

Arnica

Arnica montana

Widely used in both herbal and homeopathic medicine, arnica's vivid yellow flowers make an excellent remedy for aches and pains of all kinds.

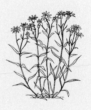

MEDICINAL USES

Part used Flower

Key actions Analgesic (relieves pain) ● Anti-inflammatory ● Wound healer

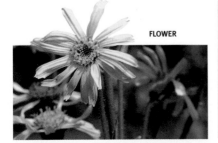

FLOWER

Injuries Quick and effective in easing bruises, sprains, and sports injuries, arnica's pain-relieving properties also make it valuable in healing wounds following an operation or dental treatment.

KEY INFORMATION

SAFETY	★ ★ ★ ★ ☆
TRADITIONAL USE	★ ★ ★ ★ ☆
RESEARCH	★ ★ ⯪ ☆ ☆

BEST TAKEN AS Lotion, cream, ointment ✓✓✓
DOSAGE Topical
CAUTIONS External use only; toxic when taken internally. Do not apply to broken skin or open wounds. See also pp.42–51.

Angelica

Angelica archangelica

The botanical name of angelica points to the highly prized status of this northern European herb in the past. A warming tonic that is good for both poor digestion and weak circulation, angelica is also an excellent remedy to support recovery from chronic illness and to revitalize a delicate digestive system.

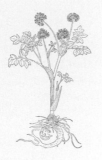

MEDICINAL USES

Parts used Root ● Seed

Key actions Expectorant ● Muscle relaxant (mild) ● Relieves gas
● Stimulates appetite and digestive juices
● Stimulates sweating and cooling
● Strengthens weak circulation

Digestive system The bitter taste of angelica— best savored as a tincture—stimulates stomach activity, making it a key remedy for poor appetite and anorexia. It soothes cramping and sensations of fullness in the digestive tract, and eases gas.

Respiratory problems Angelica eases conditions such as asthma, bronchitis, chest congestion, and cough, and is an ideal remedy for recuperation after an acute chest infection.

Found in temperate regions as far apart as western Europe, Siberia, and the Himalayas, angelica grows in damp sites.

KEY INFORMATION

SAFETY	★ ★ ★ ★ ☆
TRADITIONAL USE	★ ★ ★ ★ ☆
RESEARCH	★ ☆ ☆ ☆ ☆

BEST TAKEN AS Tincture ✓✓✓ Capsule ✓✓ Tablet ✓

DOSAGE C (*see pp.44–45*)

OFTEN USED WITH Chamomile (*Chamomilla recutita*)

CAUTIONS Do not take if pregnant or if taking anticoagulants (blood-thinning drugs). Not advisable during heavy menstrual bleeding. See also pp.42–51.

DRIED ROOT

Other uses The root's warming and stimulatory action upon the heart and circulation improves the blood flow throughout the whole body, making it useful in problems such as cold hands and feet, chilblains, and fibromyalgia.

Chinese angelica, Dong quai

Angelica sinensis

One of the most popular of all Chinese herbs, Chinese angelica is regarded as the main women's tonic, helping to support a regular menstrual cycle and easing menstrual pain. As a warming and relaxing remedy that strengthens digestive and liver activity, it is suitable for both men and women.

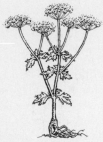

MEDICINAL USES

Part used Root

Key actions Digestive tonic ● Female reproductive tonic ● Relieves menstrual pain

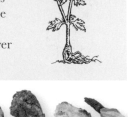

root is used as a uterine tonic

DRIED ROOT

Menstrual problems Also known as dong quai, Chinese angelica may be taken to help maintain a normal menstrual cycle or to treat menstrually linked problems such as breast tenderness and painful periods. In the case of irregular or missed periods, it will often help to establish a more regular menstrual cycle if taken for several months. However, it should be avoided during heavy menstrual bleeding. Although Chinese angelica appears to have no direct hormonal activity, it has the reputation of helping to improve fertility, combining well with chaste berry (*Vitex agnus-castus*) in this respect.

TINCTURE

Other uses A digestive tonic that promotes appetite and absorption, Chinese angelica also stimulates the circulation and protects the liver.

Pleasant-tasting and with a slightly peppery flavor, Chinese angelica is a common ingredient in Chinese medicinal food dishes.

KEY INFORMATION

SAFETY ★★★★☆
TRADITIONAL USE ★★★★★
RESEARCH ★★☆☆☆
BEST TAKEN AS Decoction ✓✓✓
Tincture ✓✓ Capsule, tablet ✓
DOSAGE C (*see pp.44–45*)
OFTEN USED WITH Chaste berry
(*Vitex agnus-castus*)
CAUTIONS Do not take during pregnancy or if taking anticoagulant (blood-thinning) medication. Not advisable during heavy menstrual bleeding. See also pp.42–51.

Celery

Apium graveolens

A good detoxification remedy, celery stem, leaf, and seed stimulate the kidneys to clear waste products, especially helping to cleanse salts that accumulate in joints, causing stiffness and inflammation. Although celery today is considered to be a mild sedative, in earlier times it was believed to be an aphrodisiac.

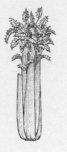

MEDICINAL USES

Parts used Leaf ● Seed ● Stem

Key actions Anti-inflammatory ● Antirheumatic ● Relieves gas ● Stimulates urine flow

Arthritic and rheumatic problems

Celery is a key remedy in European herbal medicine in the treatment of arthritic and rheumatic problems where joints, muscles, and tendons are sore, swollen, or stiff. The seed contains a volatile oil which stimulates the clearance of waste products by the kidneys. In particular, it supports the elimination of salts such as urates that often cause inflammation and stiffness within the muscular-skeletal system. Celery seed is taken to ease joint and muscle pain and stiffness, especially when it occurs in the early morning. It also clears fluid accumulation linked to arthritis. Gout is one of its main indications—the seed can be taken to relieve symptoms and prevent recurrence.

Detox remedy Juice from the stem and leaf is an excellent dietary supplement in aiding detoxification and weight loss. It is particularly suitable for people with a tendency to retain fluids.

Other uses Celery seed may also be taken to relieve gas and bloating.

KEY INFORMATION

SAFETY	★ ★ ★ ★ ☆
TRADITIONAL USE	★ ★ ★ ★ ☆
RESEARCH	★ ★ ☆ ☆ ☆

BEST TAKEN AS Tincture ✓✓✓ Capsule ✓✓ Tablet ✓
DOSAGE D (see pp.44–45)
OFTEN USED WITH Willow bark (*Salix alba*)
CAUTIONS Seeds not to be taken during pregnancy or in kidney disease. Can occasionally cause allergic reactions, including contact dermatitis. See also pp.42–51.

a nutritious vegetable

STEM AND LEAVES

seeds contain volatile oil

DRIED SEEDS

Both the juice and seed of celery stimulate urine flow and can prove useful as part of a broad approach to treating high blood pressure.

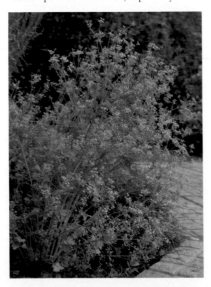

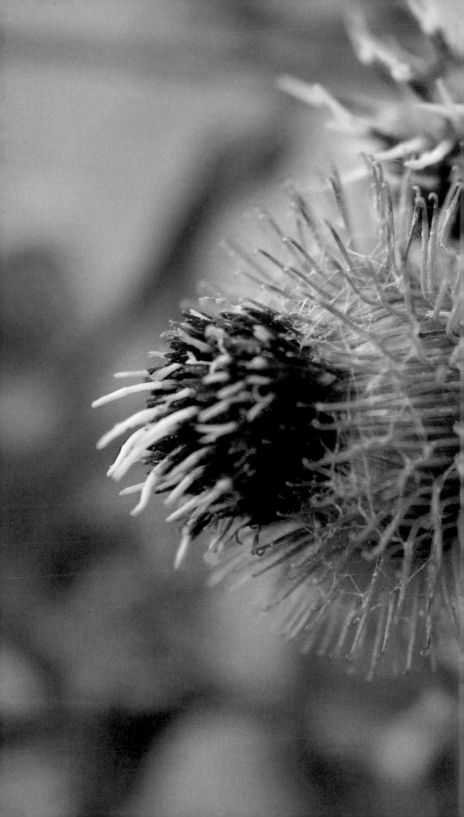

One of the foremost detoxifying herbs in Western and Chinese herbal medicine, burdock (*Arctium lappa*) is used to cleanse the body of waste products, including heavy metals.

Burdock

Arctium lappa

Traditionally combined with dandelion to make a tonic, cleansing drink, burdock is an important detox remedy in both Western and Chinese herbal traditions. Often used to treat skin problems, burdock also supports the immune system during infection and chronic illness.

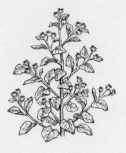

MEDICINAL USES

Parts used Root ● Seed

Key actions Antiseptic ● Detoxifying remedy ● Diuretic ● Tonic

Blood cleanser Although much undervalued, burdock may be used in any situation in which the body needs increased clearance of waste products. Conditions as varied as acne, boils, eczema, arthritis, fibromyalgia, and tonsillitis will benefit from the herb's pronounced ability to stimulate release of waste products from the cells.

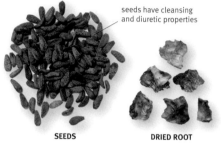

seeds have cleansing and diuretic properties

SEEDS

DRIED ROOT

KEY INFORMATION

SAFETY	★ ★ ★ ★ ☆
TRADITIONAL USE	★ ★ ★ ★ ☆
RESEARCH	★ ☆ ☆ ☆ ☆

BEST TAKEN AS Decoction ✓✓✓ Tincture ✓✓ Tablet ✓
DOSAGE A (*see pp.44–45*)
OFTEN USED WITH Yellow dock (*Rumex crispus*)
CAUTIONS Very rarely, can cause contact dermatitis. See also pp.41–52.

However, it should be used with caution as even small amounts can cause an initial flare-up in symptoms, particularly in skin disorders. For this reason, it is rarely used on its own and is combined with remedies such as dandelion (*Taraxacum officinale*), red clover (*Trifolium pratense*), and yellow dock (*Rumex crispus*) that counterbalance its detoxifying action. Although it is not yet substantiated, burdock root is thought to have marked anticancer activity.

Leaves can be used as a poultice for acne and boils.

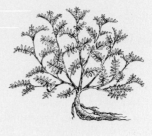

Astragalus

Astragalus membranaceus

This remarkable herb has been used in Chinese herbal medicine for over 2,000 years, and scientific research is beginning to confirm (and to some degree, extend) its range of uses. Astragalus is a safe remedy, often helpful in cases of chronic infection.

MEDICINAL USES

Part used Root

Key actions Antioxidant ● Immune support ● Tonic

Low endurance and weak immune resistance Seen as a specific remedy for supporting a weak or compromised immune system, astragalus is also classified as an adaptogen, strengthening the body's ability to cope with the physical aspects of stress. The root is used to treat many longstanding health problems, especially those that involve chronic infection, weakness, and exhaustion. Chronic fatigue syndrome, viral infections, and debility can all benefit from medium to long-term use of the herb. Astragalus

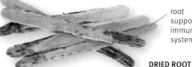

root supports immune system

DRIED ROOT

KEY INFORMATION

SAFETY	★ ★ ★ ★ ☆
TRADITIONAL USE	★ ★ ★ ★ ★
RESEARCH	★ ★ ★ ½ ☆

BEST TAKEN AS Decoction ✓✓✓ Tincture ✓✓ Capsule, tablet ✓
DOSAGE A (*see pp.44–45*)
OFTEN USED WITH Schisandra (*Schisandra chinensis*).
CAUTIONS No known side effects. Avoid in acute illness. See also pp.42–51.

also has a persistent reputation for helping to control sweating, especially where this is linked to chronic illness.

Cancer Although astragalus is not a treatment for cancer in its own right, it nevertheless has much to offer in supporting immune function and maintaining a sense of well-being. It is best taken either as a preventative or alongside conventional treatment such as chemotherapy. Clinical research suggests that astragalus reduces the toxic effects of chemotherapy and at the same time enhances immune function. The root may need to be taken long-term to achieve best results. Seek professional advice from your doctor or herbal practitioner before taking astragalus along with chemotherapy.

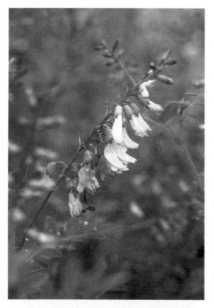

Native to China and Mongolia, astragalus is one of the most popular tonic herbs in China and is used to improve energy levels and increase endurance.

Oats

Avena sativa

Better known as a food, oats are a valuable medicinal plant that benefit the health of the nervous system. A good source of both B vitamins and vitamin E, oats are absorbed slowly into the blood stream, have a low glycemic index, and support better-balanced blood sugar levels.

MEDICINAL USES

Parts used Dried seed ● Fresh plant

Key actions Antidepressant ● Emollient ● Nutritive ● Tonic

Nervous problems Oats can be taken therapeutically to improve nervous stamina and lift depressed mood. Traditional use ascribes antidepressant activity to the dried seeds and fresh plant, and may be useful where lowered mood is associated with anxiety and nervous exhaustion, especially during menopause. The fresh plant is a tonic remedy for all types of nervous debility, and can help to improve sleep duration and quality where the person is literally too tired to sleep. Oats also aid withdrawal from tobacco and drug addiction.

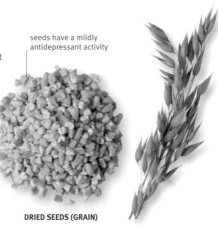

seeds have a mildly antidepressant activity

DRIED SEEDS (GRAIN)

Eczema The dried seeds can be used to make a decoction to relieve the symptoms of eczema. Put the seeds in a muslin bag under a running hot bathwater tap so that the decoction is strained into the bath—the soothing emollient activity of the seeds eases itching and nourishes the skin.

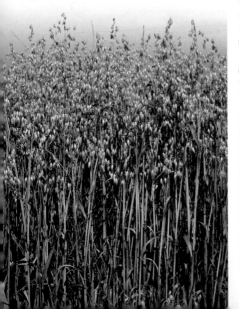

Oats are grown principally as a cereal crop. Their tonic action on the nervous system has led herbalists to describe them as a food for the nerves.

KEY INFORMATION

SAFETY	★ ★ ★ ★ ★
TRADITIONAL USE	★ ★ ★ ⯨ ☆
RESEARCH	★ ★ ⯨ ☆ ☆

BEST TAKEN AS Dried seed: Food ✓ ✓ ✓ Tincture ✓ ✓ Fresh plant: Tincture ✓ ✓ ✓ Capsule ✓ ✓

DOSAGE A (*see pp.44–45*)

OFTEN USED WITH Damiana (*Turnera diffusa*) for nervous exhaustion or stress with depressed mood.

CAUTIONS None known. See also pp.42–51.

Neem

Azadirachta indica

A large evergreen tree, neem is a veritable pharmacy in its own right, as well as a natural insecticide. The seed, seed oil, leaf, and bark are used medicinally, and have have been used in conditions as diverse as scabies and psoriasis, malaria, diabetes, and anxiety.

MEDICINAL USES

Parts used Bark ● Leaf ● Seed ● Twig

Key actions Antibacterial ● Antifungal ● Anti-inflammatory ● Blood cleanser ● Immune support ● Lowers blood sugar levels ● Relieves itchiness

Skin conditions Neem's most common use in the West is as an oil, which can bring relief to sore and itchy rashes. It may be safely applied to irritated or inflamed skin such as in eczema and psoriasis, and can be used to treat head lice, scabies, and fungal problems such as ringworm. The oil may also be applied as a poultice to boils, helping to draw out toxins.

Other uses Taken internally, neem's many uses include bacterial, fungal, and viral infection, allergic reactions such as asthma, diabetes, digestive problems such as peptic ulcers, and liver disorders. A strong-acting remedy, neem appears to be safe at normal dosage, but it is best taken internally when prescribed by an herbal practitioner or doctor. Neem has contraceptive activity and should be avoided by women who are trying to conceive.

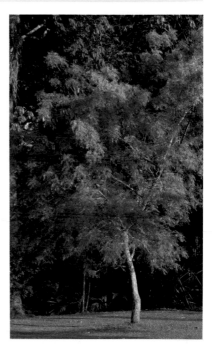

Planted in villages and towns throughout India, neem often acts as a community medicinal resource and is one of the most valued herbs in Ayurvedic medicine.

KEY INFORMATION

SAFETY	★ ★ ☆ ☆ ☆
TRADITIONAL USE	★ ★ ★ ★ ★
RESEARCH	★ ★ ★ ☆ ☆

BEST TAKEN AS Tincture ✓ ✓ ✓ Capsule ✓ ✓ Tablet ✓

DOSAGE C (*see pp.44–45*)

CAUTIONS Do not take during pregnancy, while breast-feeding, or during fertility treatment. In children, use topically *only*. Keep to recommended dosage—long-term high-dose use is not advisable. See also pp.42–51.

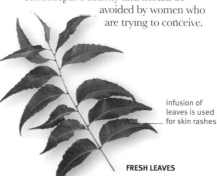

infusion of leaves is used for skin rashes

FRESH LEAVES

Bacopa

Bacopa monniera

An important Ayurvedic herb, bacopa is known for reducing nervous overactivity and improving mental performance.

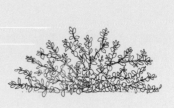

MEDICINAL USES

Part used Dried whole plant

Key actions Mild analgesic ● Mild sedative ● Nerve tonic

KEY INFORMATION

SAFETY   ★ ★ ★ ★ ☆
TRADITIONAL USE ★ ★ ★ ★ ★
RESEARCH   ★ ★ ⯪ ☆ ☆
BEST TAKEN AS Capsule ✓✓✓ Tablet ✓✓ Tincture ✓
DOSAGE B (*see pp.44–45*)
CAUTIONS Can cause digestive irritation. See also pp.42–51.

Nervous and digestive disorders

A gentle-acting remedy for nervous exhaustion, anxiety, and stress, bacopa also benefits digestion by cooling excess heat and stimulating appetite. Traditional usage and scientific research suggest that bacopa can help to enhance memory and concentration. It also appears to improve learning ability.

WHOLE PLANT

Wild indigo root

Baptisia tinctoria

A Native American herb used to cleanse wounds and counter infection, wild indigo has been used with echinacea to treat acute infection.

MEDICINAL USES

Part used Root

KEY INFORMATION

SAFETY   ★ ★ ★ ☆ ☆
TRADITIONAL USE ★ ★ ★ ★ ☆
RESEARCH   ★ ☆ ☆ ☆ ☆
BEST TAKEN AS Tincture ✓✓✓ Capsule ✓✓
DOSAGE C (*see pp.44–45*)
OFTEN USED WITH Echinacea (*Echinacea* spp.)
CAUTIONS Do not take during pregnancy and while breast-feeding. Take for a maximum of 1 week at a time unless advised by a herbal or medical practitioner. Can occasionally cause nausea and vomiting. See also pp.42–51.

Key actions Antimicrobial ● Detoxifying ● Immune stimulant

Bacterial infection

In throat infections, the diluted tincture may be used first as a gargle, and then swallowed. Wild indigo can prove helpful in treating a wide range of bacterial conditions, including acne, boils, and abscesses.

HERB

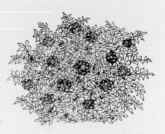

Oregon grape

Berberis aquifolium syn. *Mahonia aquifolium*

A strongly bitter-tasting herb from the Pacific northwest, Oregon grape has a long history as a digestive tonic and appetite stimulant. Over the last 20 years, evidence that supports its use in treating chronic skin disorders has grown.

MEDICINAL USES

Part used Root

Key actions Bitter tonic • Mild laxative • Skin cleanser

Digestive disorders Like its close relative, barberry (*Berberis vulgaris*), Oregon grape exerts a directly positive effect on the digestive system—inflammatory problems within the stomach or gall bladder, poor appetite, and indigestion are key indications for the herb.

Skin conditions Oregon grape is most commonly used to treat chronic inflammatory or infected skin conditions such as acne, eczema, and psoriasis. The herb contains constituents known to slow down excessive skin growth and to have antibacterial and antifungal activity. Clinical trials have found that Oregon grape extract, cream, or ointment help to relieve psoriasis. Best results are likely to be obtained by using Oregon grape in combination with other remedies that have established activity in treating chronic skin disorders.

DRIED ROOT

KEY INFORMATION

SAFETY ★ ★ ★ ⯪ ☆
TRADITIONAL USE ★ ★ ★ ☆ ☆
RESEARCH ★ ★ ★ ⯪ ☆
BEST TAKEN AS Tincture ✓✓✓
Decoction ✓✓ Capsule ✓
DOSAGE B (*see pp.44–45*)
OFTEN USED WITH Licorice (*Glycyrrhiza glabra*)
CAUTIONS Do not take during pregnancy and while breast-feeding. See also pp.42–51.

Abundant in Oregon and northern California, Oregon grape grows at high altitudes in both the Rocky Mountains and the Pacific coastal regions.

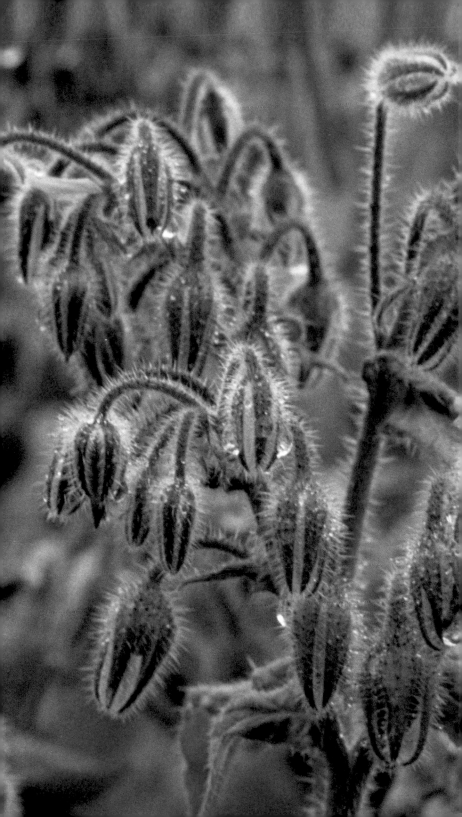

A Mediterranean plant from Spain and Morocco, borage *(Borago officinalis)* is not only grown as a garden herb and decorative plant—it is also extensively cultivated for its seed oil.

Buchu

Barosma betulina

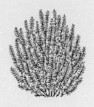

A key tonic, antiseptic, and mild stimulant herb in South African traditional medicine, buchu helps relieve urinary tract infections and gas.

MEDICINAL USES

Part used Leaf

Key action Urinary antiseptic

Urinary tract infection Buchu is used specifically for cystitis and infection in the urinary tract as a whole, since its essential oil has marked antiseptic activity. The herb is best taken as an infusion and is probably most effective when used short-

leaves contain antiseptic volatile oil

DRIED LEAVES

term for acute infections. Other herbs such as cranberry (*Vaccinium macrocarpon*) may be better for chronic conditions.

KEY INFORMATION

SAFETY ★★★★☆
TRADITIONAL USE ★★★★⯪
RESEARCH ★☆☆☆☆
BEST TAKEN AS Infusion ✓✓✓ Tincture ✓✓ Capsule ✓
DOSAGE B (*see pp.44–45*)
OFTEN USED WITH Corn silk (*Zea mays*)
  CAUTIONS During pregnancy, take only on the recommendation of an herbal or medical practitioner. Potentially toxic at excess dosage. See also pp.42–51.

Borage, Starflower

Borago officinalis

A native European and north African annual, borage seed—with up to 25% oil content—is widely used as a source of omega-6 fatty acids.

MEDICINAL USES

Part used Seed oil

KEY INFORMATION

SAFETY ★★★★★
TRADITIONAL USE ★★☆☆☆
RESEARCH ★★★★☆
BEST TAKEN AS Oil ✓✓✓ Capsule ✓✓
DOSAGE M (*see pp.44–45*)
CAUTIONS Seed oil: best taken with food. Seek advice from an herbal or medical practitioner if taking epilepsy medication. Avoid other borage products, which are thought to contain constituents that are potentially toxic to the liver. See also pp.42–51.

Key actions Anti-inflammatory ● Antioxidant ● Emollient (soothes skin)

Chronic skin disorders With its high omega-6 fatty acid content, borage oil has significant anti-inflammatory activity, and taken over several months can improve skin conditions such as eczema. Apply locally to dry or itchy skin patches.

FLOWERS

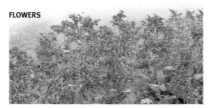

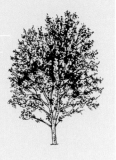

Birch

Betula alba

The birch tree has a long history of use in northern temperate regions of the world. Birch tar oil, distilled from the bark, is a traditional treatment for chronic skin diseases. The leaves are used in kidney and rheumatic disorders, and the sap, tapped early spring, is taken as a refreshing and cleansing tonic.

MEDICINAL USES

Parts used Bark ● Leaf

Key actions Anti-inflammatory
● Astringent ● Diuretic ● Mild analgesic
● Stimulates sweating

Rheumatic and kidney problems

Birch's unusual combination of actions makes it a valuable remedy in conditions where symptoms reflecting kidney weakness—poor urine output, fluid retention, and puffiness—occur side by side with rheumatic problems such as stiff and aching problems, arthritic pain, and leg cramps. By aiding the clearance of waste products in urine, birch leaves increase the body's ability to remove waste products from joint and muscle tissues. The leaves contain aspirin-like substances which contribute to their ability to control inflammation and relieve pain. Traditional uses of birch include rheumatic pain, gout, fibromyalgia, and kidney and urinary tract infections such as cystitis. A warm decoction of the leaves and twigs can be applied to ease stiff and aching muscles. The sap is thought to have diuretic properties.

Few trees have proved to be more useful than the birch: in addition to its medicinal qualities, the bark is used as tinder and paper, and the trunk is made into buckets and canoes.

KEY INFORMATION

SAFETY ★ ★ ★ ★ ☆
TRADITIONAL USE ★ ★ ★ ☆ ☆
RESEARCH ★ ★ ☆ ☆ ☆
BEST TAKEN AS Infusion ✓✓✓ Tincture ✓✓
Capsule ✓
DOSAGE A (see pp.44–45)
OFTEN USED WITH Willow bark (Salix alba)
CAUTIONS None known.
See also pp.41–52.

DRIED LEAVES

Other uses A favorite Scandinavian remedy, birch twig bundles are used in saunas and steam baths to penetrate the skin and muscles in order to stimulate sweating, invigorate, and relieve tender and aching muscles. Birch oil, extracted from the leaves and twigs, is a traditional northern European product, commonly used in external applications for rheumatic aches and pains.

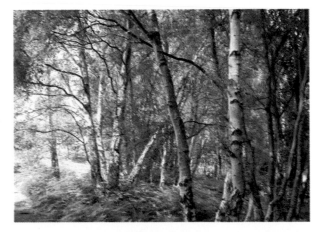

Boswellia

Boswellia serrata

Boswellia is highly prized in traditional Indian medicine and has been used to treat conditions as varied as arthritis, asthma, bronchitis, dysentery, and fever. The rationale for its traditional use has been largely confirmed by recent scientific research.

MEDICINAL USES

Part used Resin

Key actions Anti-inflammatory
● Anti-arthritic ● Antiseptic
● Reduces fever

Arthritic problems Boswellia is fast becoming one of the most commonly taken medicines for arthritic problems. Concerns over the safety of conventional anti-inflammatories have increased interest in herbal alternatives, and in boswellia's case, there is a significant and growing body of research that indicates both its safety and effectiveness. The specific anti-inflammatory action of the resin makes it an important remedy for chronic inflammatory conditions such as rheumatoid arthritis and gout. It can also prove valuable in relieving pain and stiffness in osteoarthritis.

Other uses Boswellia is also indicated in other inflammatory conditions such as asthma, ulcerative colitis, and multiple sclerosis. It has recently been used to treat brain tumors and Alzheimer's disease—in both cases, it should be used only under professional supervision.

Boswellia is a relative of frankincense (*Boswellia sacra*), and is sometimes known as Indian frankincense. It grows in India and North Africa.

resin is antiseptic

KEY INFORMATION

SAFETY	★ ★ ★ ★ ☆
TRADITIONAL USE	★ ★ ★ ★ ☆
RESEARCH	★ ★ ★ ★ ☆

BEST TAKEN AS Tablet: standardized to 60% boswellic acid content ✓✓✓
DOSAGE M (*see pp.44–45*)
OFTEN USED WITH Ginger (*Zingiber officinalis*)
CAUTIONS Can cause contact dermatitis. See also pp.42–51.

standardized extract in tablet form

TABLETS

Bupleurum, Chai hu

Bupleurum falcatum, B. chinensis

A member of the carrot family, bupleurum root is a commonly used remedy in China and Japan, its main traditional applications being flu, flu colds and fever, irregular menstrual cycle, and liver disorders. It is a good bitter-tasting tonic and, as with all bitter remedies, stimulates appetite and digestive function.

MEDICINAL USES

Part used Root

Key actions Anti-inflammatory
● Bitter tonic ● Protects liver
● Stimulates sweating

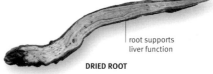

root supports
liver function

DRIED ROOT

Immune function Ongoing research over the last 30 years—mostly in Japan— suggests that bupleurum has a unique combination of medicinal benefits. It has potent anti-inflammatory activity, similar in some ways to steroid medication, which helps reduce and prevent inflammation throughout the body. At the same time, bupleurum enhances immune function and protects both liver and kidneys from damage. Its key use is therefore in liver and kidney disorders, especially where these are under stress due to chronic inflammation, toxicity, or autoimmune disease. It may be safely self-medicated for straightforward health problems, for example in treating colds, flu, and fever, but should be taken only on professional recommendation in serious illness such as autoimmune disease.

KEY INFORMATION

SAFETY	★★★★☆
TRADITIONAL USE	★★★★★
RESEARCH	★★★☆☆

BEST TAKEN AS Decoction ✓✓✓
Tincture ✓✓ Tablet ✓
DOSAGE B (*see pp.44–45*)
OFTEN USED WITH Astragalus
(*Astragalus membranaceus*)
CAUTIONS Can occasionally cause gastrointestinal symptoms such as flatulence, nausea, and vomiting.
See also pp.42–51.

DECOCTION

Other uses In traditional Chinese medicine, bupleurum is combined with herbs such as white peony (*Paeonia lactiflora*) and licorice (*Glycyrrhiza glabra*) to treat conditions such as irregular menstrual activity and prolapsed womb.

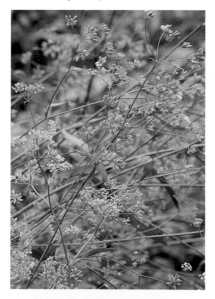

Buplureum's use in China as a liver tonic extends back at least 2,000 years. The root is dug up in spring or autumn when it contains the most active constituents.

Difficult to mistake for any other plant, calendula (*Calendula officinalis*) is instantly recognized by its bright orange flower heads. The flowers are used to heal rashes and inflamed skin.

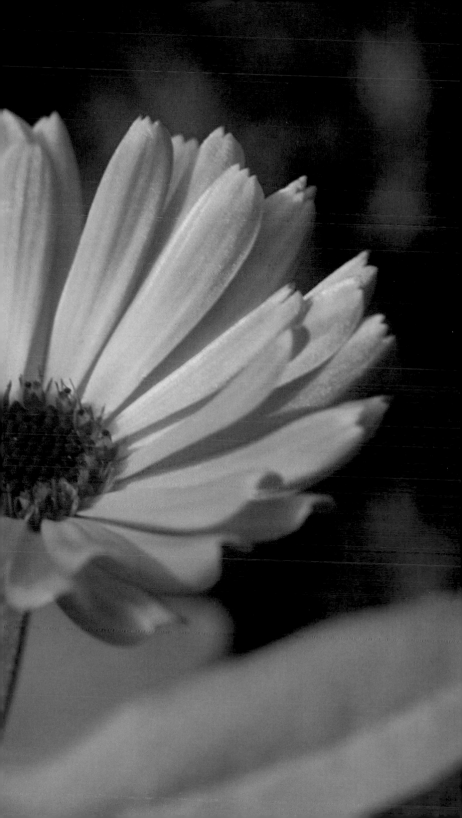

Marigold, Calendula

Calendula officinalis

Calendula is best known as a cream or ointment that makes a soothing and healing application to sore, angry, or inflamed skin. The herb's bright orange flower heads can also be prepared as an infusion that, once cooled, makes a soothing wash or lotion for hot and inflamed rashes, cuts, or grazes.

MEDICINAL USES

Part used Flower

Key actions Antifungal
- Anti-inflammatory ● Antimicrobial
- Blood cleanser ● Wound healer

Skin infections Whether applied topically on the skin or taken internally, calendula has antiseptic, cleansing, and detoxifying properties, and a wealth of potential uses. As a lotion, cream, or ointment, it will speed healing and counter infection in conditions as diverse as minor burns and sunburn, insect bites and stings, sore and pustular spots, mastitis, cuts and abrasions, inflamed rashes, hemorrhoids, and varicose veins.

Digestive disorders Taken internally (best as an infusion), calendula may be used to help heal inflammatory problems throughout the digestive tract, including peptic ulcers

AERIAL PARTS

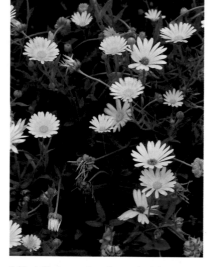

Cultivated in temperate regions, calendula grows well in almost all soils. The flowers are harvested in early summer when they open.

and gastritis. Due in part to its antifungal properties, it will aid recovery from gastrointestinal infection, especially when linked to gut dysbiosis and candidiasis, and help to treat problems such as acne, throat infections, and mastitis. As an infusion, it combines well with herbs such as cleavers (*Galium aparine*), red clover (*Trifolium pratense*), and chamomile (*Chamomilla recutita*).

KEY INFORMATION

SAFETY	★ ★ ★ ★ ☆
TRADITIONAL USE	★ ★ ★ ★ ☆
RESEARCH	★ ★ ⯪ ☆ ☆

BEST TAKEN AS Infusion ✓✓✓ Tincture ✓✓
Capsule ✓
DOSAGE B (*see pp.44–45*)
OFTEN USED WITH Cleavers (*Galium aparine*)
CAUTIONS Can occasionally cause allergic reactions. See also pp.42–51.

flowers have antiseptic properties

DRIED FLOWERS

Senna

Cassia spp.

A well-known herb, senna grows in much of North Africa, the Middle East, and India, and its use has become almost universal. It was first used by Arab physicians in the 9th century CE. With its strong laxative action, senna makes an effective short-term treatment for constipation.

MEDICINAL USES

Parts used Leaf • Pod

Key actions Stimulant laxative

Constipation Senna is primarily used to treat acute and short-term constipation—and it usually achieves this end efficiently. Senna is best taken in the evening, as active constituents within both leaf and pod irritate the muscles of the colon and normally result in a bowel movement 6–8 hours later. The standard advice is to take senna for up to a maximum of two weeks at a time. If constipation remains a problem after two weeks, seek advice from your herbal practitioner or doctor. To minimize the chances of griping, senna should be combined with a relaxant remedy such as chamomile (*Chamomilla recutita*), fennel (*Foeniculum vulgare*), or ginger (*Zingiber officinalis*). At the appropriate dosage, senna is a very safe medicine. Not only is it safe to take during pregnancy and while breast-feeding, but it seems to be the laxative of choice to relieve the constipation that commonly occurs during pregnancy.

KEY INFORMATION

SAFETY	★ ★ ★ ★ ☆
TRADITIONAL USE	★ ★ ★ ★ ★
RESEARCH	★ ★ ★ ★ ★

BEST TAKEN AS Tablet ✓✓✓ Syrup ✓✓
DOSAGE M (*see pp.44–45*)
OFTEN USED WITH Ginger (*Zingiber officinalis*)
CAUTIONS Take at recommended dosage only—may cause abdominal cramping. See also pp.42–51.

Native to Africa, senna is a small shrub with a woody stem.

milder in effect than leaves

used in tablets to treat constipation

DRIED PODS

Tea

Camellia sinensis

Grown almost exclusively for use as a beverage, tea is perhaps the world's most undervalued medicinal plant. Numerous studies point to the health-giving properties of the tea leaf, especially unfermented green or white tea. These teas contain high levels of polyphenols, which have potent antioxidant activity.

MEDICINAL USES

Parts used Leaf bud ● Young leaf

Key actions Antioxidant ● Astringent ● Diuretic ● Stimulant

Stimulant Traditionally, tea has been seen as a gentle stimulant, its moderate caffeine content enhancing mental alertness and acting as a "pick-me-up." Like coffee (*Coffea arabica*), it has been used as a remedy for headache, although coffee is probably more effective in this respect. Tea has warming and tonic properties, endearing it to those working in the cold. It is best avoided during premenstrual syndrome—research has repeatedly shown that caffeine leads to a worsening of symptoms, and may be unhelpful during menopause, as it can increase hot flashes.

Digestive problems As an astringent, tea makes a useful and readily available remedy for diarrhea; the polyphenols in the tea counter infection and tone up the inner lining of the gut. In

green tea prevents tooth decay

FRESH LEAVES

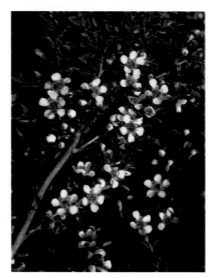

Recent studies suggest that the polyphenolic compounds in tea may promote fertility in women who drink one to two cups daily.promotes fertility.

combination with other remedies, traditional Chinese medicine uses tea to treat diarrhea and dysentery.

Eye problems For tired, irritated, and puffy eyes, place a moist tea bag or a cotton ball that has been soaked in cooled green tea on the affected (closed) eye for a few minutes. Usually symptoms are eased and the eyelids and surrounding tissues are toned. Tea can also be used in this way to counter inflammation or

brew of tea leaves soothes sunburn

DRIED LEAVES

KEY INFORMATION

SAFETY	★ ★ ★ ★ ★
TRADITIONAL USE	★ ★ ★ ★ ☆
RESEARCH	★ ★ ★ ★ ☆

BEST TAKEN AS Infusion ✓✓✓
Tablet ✓✓ Capsule ✓
DOSAGE B (*see pp.44–45*)
CAUTIONS Avoid excessive doses.
See also pp.42–51.

infection within the eye, for example, in helping to relieve the pain and discomfort of conjunctivitis.

Other uses Recent research has focused on the antioxidant polyphenols, which have been found to aid weight loss, to counter inflammation, and to have anticancer and antitumor activity. The high intake of green tea in China and Japan is thought to be partly responsible for the low incidence of cancer in these countries. Tea also appears to reduce the incidence of tooth decay. Not surprisingly, green tea has become a popular drink in the West in recent years, although it is worth noting that research suggests that tea impairs absorption of iron and other minerals. Avoid drinking tea with meals or medication, especially if anemic.

Tea quality Green tea is produced by lightly steaming the freshly cut bud and leaf, leaving the active constituents largely intact. However, black tea is allowed to ferment,

GREEN TEA

Tea is cultivated mainly in India, Sri Lanka, and China. Tea leaves are picked throughout the year.

AGE-OLD BREW

One of the legends surrounding tea drinking features Shen Nung, a 3rd-century BCE Chinese emperor. It is said that as he sat under a tree, boiling his drinking water, a few leaves from the tree (*Camellia sinensis*) fell into his kettle. Shen Nung drank the brew and found the taste quite agreeable, thus prompting the longstanding tradition of tea drinking.

TEA CADDY

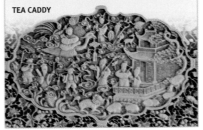

leading to a significant loss of antioxidant constituents, notably polyphenols. High-quality teas—such as white or Oolong tea, which is made with the youngest leaf buds— have the highest levels of polyphenols, and can be expensive, although not as costly as in the 18th century, when the finest teas were literally worth their weight in gold.

Chili, Cayenne pepper

Capsicum spp.

Familiar the world over, chili comes from the Americas, and its strongly pungent flavor spices up countless dishes. The constituents responsible for the hot, sometimes fiercely hot, impact of chili when eaten are also those most involved in its many medicinal applications.

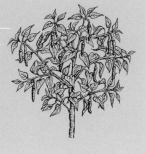

MEDICINAL USES

Part used Fruit

Key actions Antiseptic ● Local analgesic ● Counterirritant ● Relieves gas and spasm ● Stimulant ● Tonic

Circulation When it is applied to the skin as a counterirritant, chili, like other hot, pungent remedies such as mustard (*Sinapsis alba*), causes irritation and swelling, and an increase in circulation to the area. Chili is added to lotions, liniments, and salves for muscular aches and pains for this reason, resulting in better nutrition to—and clearance of waste products from—the tissue involved.

Nerve pain Chili peppers are graded according to their "heat"; the hotter the taste, the higher the level of capsaicin— the key active constituent present within the flesh of the pepper. Capsaicin initially increases the awareness of pain and inflammation, but then desensitizes the local nerve endings, leading to reduced levels of pain. This action is utilized in capsaicin creams for conditions such as post-herpetic neuralgia (shingles), nerve pain linked to diabetes, and also for severe itchiness. These products are often only available with a prescription.

Introduced to Europe in the 16th century, chili is now cultivated throughout the tropics.

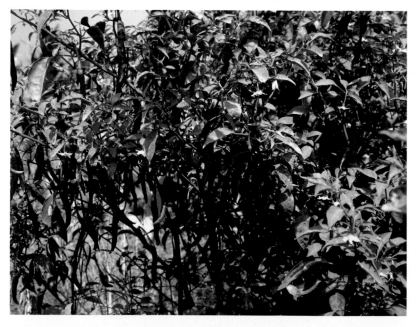

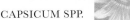

General stimulant Rarely used on its own, chili is most commonly added to other herbs to strengthen and stimulate their action within the body. Adding small quantities of chili powder, sauce, or tincture can provide an important boost to the effects of an herbal mixture. For example, a few drops of chili sauce or tincture can be mixed with echinacea (*Echinacea* spp.) and licorice (*Glycyrrhiza glabra*) tincture to treat throat infection. To strengthen the circulation and to improve blood flow to hands and feet, small quantities of chili can be routinely added to food. Chili also mixes well with specific remedies such as devil's claw (*Harpagophytum procumbens*) when treating conditions such as osteoarthritis and fibromyalgia, where circulation to affected areas is often poor. Chili's general stimulant effect also finds use where the thyroid gland is mildly underactive. Here, chili will help to strengthen the circulation and improve metabolic rate. Recent research points to the possibility that chili works to enhance the anticancer activity of other antioxidant remedies. Although data is based so far only on test tube research, scientists found that when they combined 1 part chili preparation with 25 parts green tea concentrate, the anticancer activity of the combination was 100 times greater than the green tea alone. This suggests that chili can have a major impact on the medicinal activity of other foods and herbal remedies.

KEY INFORMATION

SAFETY	★ ★ ★ ★ ☆
TRADITIONAL USE	★ ★ ★ ★ ★
RESEARCH	★ ★ ★ ☆ ☆

BEST TAKEN AS Capsule ✓✓✓
DOSAGE C (*see pp.44–45*)
CAUTIONS Non-toxic at normal dose; caution required when eating or handling hot chili products. Can cause intense pain and burning, and contact dermatitis. See also pp.42–51.

CHILI POWDER

Weak digestive system Chili has antiseptic properties and helps to protect against gastrointestinal infection. It is often added to food in tropical countries to reduce the risk of food poisoning. Used in small quantities, chili will help to strengthen a weak digestive system and stimulate appetite, particularly in older people, though it can benefit anyone with an under-performing digestive system. A pinch of chili powder added to chamomile (*Chamomilla recutita*) tea or tincture will help to relieve nausea and feelings of fullness. Surprisingly, chili can be an effective remedy for treating diarrhea.

CHILI "PEPPER"

Chili was one of many medicinal plants Christopher Columbus brought back from the New World to present to his patrons, the Spanish king and queen. The hot taste of chili, similar to that of black pepper from Indonesia, encouraged Columbus to call it chili "pepper," thereby suggesting that it also came from eastern Asia, and that his mission to find a western route to the East Indies had been successful.

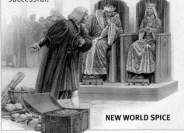

NEW WORLD SPICE

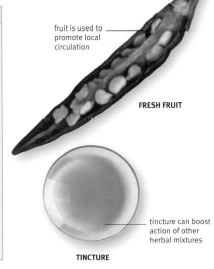

fruit is used to promote local circulation

FRESH FRUIT

tincture can boost action of other herbal mixtures

TINCTURE

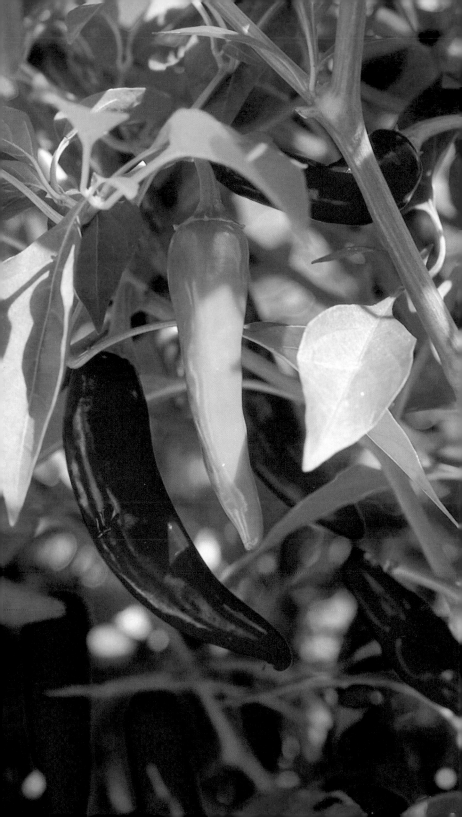

The hot taste of chili (*Capsicum* spp.) points toward its medicinal use as a powerful warming stimulant. A popular ingredient in Mexican cuisine, it has even been used to flavor ice cream.

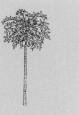

Papaya, Paw paw

Carica papaya

A sweet-tasting fruit and native to tropical America, papaya while unripe contains digestive enzymes that complement the body's own digestive juices.

MEDICINAL USES

Parts used Fruit pulp ● Latex (extract)

Key actions Digestive ● Nutritive

Digestive problems When the unripe fruit is cut, a thick white juice or latex containing papain (digestive enzyme) seeps out. Papain breaks down protein, especially in an alkaline environment, making it a useful supplement that promotes effective digestion within the small intestine, in particular when normal digestive secretions are deficient. Papain is also used as a food tenderizer, especially in the fast food industry.

Other uses The ripe fruit is nutritious, cleansing, and mildly laxative. Papaya seeds can be used to treat worms.

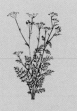

RIPE FRUIT

KEY INFORMATION

SAFETY	★ ★ ★ ★ ★
TRADITIONAL USE	★ ★ ★ ☆ ☆
RESEARCH	★ ★ ★ ☆ ☆

BEST TAKEN AS Extract: Tablet, capsule ✓✓✓
DOSAGE M – extract (*see pp.44–45*)
CAUTIONS Caution required during pregnancy when using concentrated forms of the papaya enzyme, papain. See also pp.42–51.

Caraway

Carum carvi

Used in food and medicine for at least 5,000 years, caraway is one of Europe's most popular herbs. The volatile oil in the seeds gives caraway its distinctive aroma.

MEDICINAL USES

Parts used Essential oil ● Seed

Key actions Eases coughing ● Relieves gas and spasm

KEY INFORMATION

SAFETY	★ ★ ★ ★ ☆
TRADITIONAL USE	★ ★ ★ ★ ☆
RESEARCH	★ ★ ★ ☆ ☆

BEST TAKEN AS Infusion ✓✓✓
Tincture ✓✓ Capsule ✓
DOSAGE C (*see pp.44–45*)
CAUTIONS Safe at normal dosage. See also pp.42–51.

Cramps and chronic cough Caraway's gently warming and relaxing action within the gut makes it an excellent remedy for soothing digestive problems such as nausea, indigestion, gas, and bloating. Caraway is an effective remedy for colic in children. A common ingredient in cough mixtures, it can be taken to relieve croup and chronic cough. Do not take the essential oil internally unless on professional advice.

a safe remedy for children

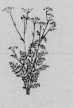

FRESH LEAVES

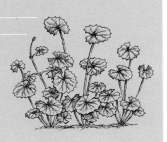

Gotu kola

Centella asiatica syn. *Hydrocotyle asiatica*

An ancient medicine, gotu kola has been in continuous use in India for at least 2,000 years. Traditionally thought to strengthen memory and concentration, in the West it is mostly used to treat chronic skin disorders and support wound healing.

MEDICINAL USES

Part used Whole plant

Key actions Adaptogen
● Anti-inflammatory ● Tonic
● Wound healer

Wounds and broken tissue Gotu kola has many potential uses, the majority revolving around its ability to promote effective tissue repair and wound healing. It speeds healing and reduces the risk of scar (or keloid) formation. Its traditional use as a treatment for leprosy reflects the herb's ability to stimulate repair of damaged tissue. It may be applied as a lotion to the skin to treat, for example, minor burns, psoriasis, and scars.

Other uses Taken internally, gotu kola appears to tone and strengthen veins, and is commonly prescribed for leg ulcers, venous insufficiency, and varicose and thread veins. As a background treatment,

A small creeping plant, gotu kola grows in the wild throughout India.

KEY INFORMATION

SAFETY ★★★★☆
TRADITIONAL USE ★★★★☆
RESEARCH ★★★☆☆
BEST TAKEN AS Tincture ✓✓✓ Tablet ✓✓
Lotion (topical) ✓
DOSAGE B (see pp.44–45)
CAUTIONS Can cause allergic reaction. Rarely, may cause gastric irritation. See also pp.42–51.

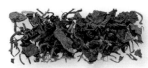

DRIED HERB

it proves useful in many chronic health problems. Its adaptogenic properties enhance the body's ability to respond to both physical and emotional stress.

plant is used to stimulate tissue healing

Helonias, False unicorn root

Chamaelirium luteum, Veratrum luteum

Used by Native American women, helonias was made popular in the 19th century by eclectic doctors in the US, trained in herbal and conventional medicine.

MEDICINAL USES

Part used Root

Key actions Estrogenic ● Uterine tonic

KEY INFORMATION

SAFETY ★★★★☆
TRADITIONAL USE ★★★★☆
RESEARCH ★☆☆☆☆
BEST TAKEN AS Organic tincture ✓✓✓
Tablet ✓✓ Capsule ✓
DOSAGE C (see pp.44–45)
CAUTIONS If pregnant, consult an herbal or medical practitioner before using. See also pp.42–51.

Women's health Despite a lack of research, helonias is a valued remedy for gynecological problems, especially those affecting the ovaries and womb. Ovarian cysts, hormonal imbalance, low fertility, and menopausal symptoms are key indications. It is an endangered plant in the wild; only organic products should be used.

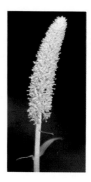

FLOWER CLUSTER

Codonopsis, Dang shen

Codonopsis pilosula

One of the many remarkable tonic remedies used within Chinese herbal medicine, codonopsis has gentle life-enhancing properties similar to ginseng.

MEDICINAL USES

Part used Root

Key actions Adaptogen ● Stimulant ● Tonic

Adaptogen Codonopsis' foremost use is for people who find ginseng too stimulating a medicine, its adaptogenic action being shorter-lasting and less fiery. It also has immune-stimulating properties.

FLOWER

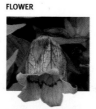

Chronic anemia Codonopsis helps to increase hemoglobin and red blood cell levels and can be a valuable remedy to take in cases of chronic anemia.

Breast-feeding In China, codonopsis is taken by nursing mothers to stimulate breast milk production.

KEY INFORMATION

SAFETY ★★★★☆
TRADITIONAL USE ★★★★☆
RESEARCH ★★☆☆☆
BEST TAKEN AS Tincture ✓✓✓
Decoction ✓✓ Tablet ✓
DOSAGE B (see pp.44–45)
CAUTIONS None known. See also pp.42–51.

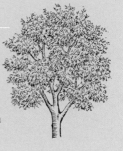

Cinnamon

Cinnamomum verum

An ancient spice, the inner bark of cinnamon leaves a pleasant and warm taste on the tongue. Its undoubted health benefits are not that well known. Recent research points to an entirely new use for it—cinnamon appears to work with insulin to help stabilize blood sugar levels in the body.

MEDICINAL USES

Parts used Essential oil ● Inner bark

Key actions Antimicrobial ● Aromatic ● Astringent ● Mild stimulant ● Relieves gas

Digestive upsets and colds Cinnamon's warming, stimulant action has made it a favorite remedy for digestive upsets. As an infusion, it helps to soothe gas, bloating, nausea, and indigestion, as well as speed recovery from gastrointestinal infection. It has moderate antibacterial and antifungal activity, and acts against *Heliobacter pylori*, an organism that can cause stomach ulcers. In colds, flu, chest infection, and coughs, cinnamon provides a pleasant treatment that can be safely given to children.

Other uses Cinnamon's ability to stimulate the circulation is often overlooked; taken long-term, it strengthens blood flow to the hands and feet, helping those with poor peripheral circulation. It can also be taken on a regular basis—one recommendation is a teaspoon of cinnamon powder at night—to support stable blood sugar levels.

KEY INFORMATION

SAFETY	★ ★ ★ ★ ☆
TRADITIONAL USE	★ ★ ★ ★ ☆
RESEARCH	★ ★ ☆ ☆ ☆

BEST TAKEN AS Infusion ✓✓✓ Tincture ✓✓ Capsule, powder ✓
DOSAGE C (*see pp.44–45*)
CAUTIONS Rarely, can cause allergic reactions. See also pp.42–51.

Native to India and Sri Lanka, cinnamon is widely cultivated as a spice and medicine.

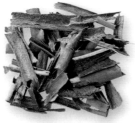

INNER BARK

German Chamomile

Chamomilla recutita syn. *Matricaria recutita*

Known more as a pleasant-tasting tea than as a medicine, chamomile provides effective treatment for health problems as diverse as indigestion and acidity, travel sickness, cramps, inflamed skin, and poor sleep. Make sure to use good-quality chamomile to achieve the best results.

MEDICINAL USES

Parts used Flower ● Essential oil

Key actions Anti-allergenic
● Anti-inflammatory ● Relaxant
● Relieves spasm ● Soothes digestion
● Wound healer

Digestive and inflammatory conditions

Perhaps the most commonly used European herb, chamomile can be safely taken by babies, children, and adults for all manner of problems affecting the digestive system. From mouth ulcers and stomach ache to colic and looseness, chamomile will soothe inflammation, acidity, and cramps and encourage effective recovery. Regular cups of chamomile tea can make a difference in inflammatory conditions such as gastritis, Crohn's disease, and colitis. For best results, brew chamomile in a teapot or in a cup with the saucer on top because most of the active

essential oil is used to treat skin problems

ESSENTIAL OIL

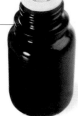

constituents are formed in the steam. Chamomile is an excellent anti-inflammatory when applied topically—use the infusion as a lotion on sore and itchy rashes, grazes, and insect bites and stings. Apply a warm chamomile teabag to sore or irritated eyes. As a lotion or poultice, the flowers can prove helpful in treating sore nipples and mastitis.

Menstrual pain and cramps The use of chamomile tea to relieve period pains and cramps predates Roman times. While other herbs may be as good or better in this respect, the ready availability of chamomile makes it an easy herb to select at the time of need.

Nervous tension Chamomile will serve well in treating other types of cramp, particularly muscle tension resulting from tension or overwork. As a mild sedative and relaxant, it can help to ease anxiety and nervous stress that interferes with normal digestive function, for example, in irritable bowel syndrome. In those prone to nervous tension and cold hands and feet, chamomile combined with ginger (*Zingiber officinalis*)—grate fresh root into a teapot—can help if taken regularly.

poultice of flower heads can relieve sore skin

DRIED FLOWER HEADS

KEY INFORMATION

SAFETY   ★ ★ ★ ★ ☆
TRADITIONAL USE   ★ ★ ★ ★ ★
RESEARCH   ★ ★ ★ ★ ☆
BEST TAKEN AS Infusion ✓✓✓ Tincture ✓✓
Essential oil (topically) ✓
DOSAGE A (*see pp.44–45*)
OFTEN USED WITH Meadowsweet
(*Filipendula ulmaria*)
CAUTIONS Rarely, can cause allergic reaction. See also pp.42–51.

Children's ailments A first-rate remedy for children, chamomile can be safely given to infants and children from the age of six months upward. In babies suffering from colic and digestive discomfort, breast-feeding mothers can drink the tea, or add a small cup of chamomile tea to the baby's bath. It soothes fussy and over-tired infants, gently encouraging relaxation and a good night's sleep. Chamomile can be confidently given to children in all gastrointestinal complaints. The tea can bring relief during teething. If taste is a problem, mix the tea with unsweetened apple or blackcurrant juice. Do not take the essential oil internally unless recommended by a professional.

A GARDENER'S DELIGHT

In medieval times, chamomile was thought of as the "plant's physician." It has been stated that nothing contributes as much to the health of a garden as chamomile herbs dispersed about it. A drooping or sickly plant may well recover if chamomile is placed near it.

GARDEN HERB

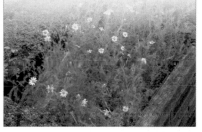

Found wild throughout Europe and temperate Asia, chamomile has also been naturalized in Australia and the US.

flower heads are used fresh or dried

Black cohosh

Cimicifuga racemosa syn. *Actaea racemosa*

Recent interest in black cohosh as an alternative to hormone replacement therapy (HRT) has led to a dramatic increase in its popularity, especially as a treatment for menopausal symptoms. A Native American remedy, black cohosh has always been seen as a herb for women's ailments.

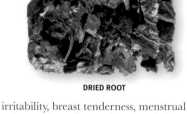

MEDICINAL USES

Part used Root

Key actions Anti-inflammatory
● Antirheumatic ● Hormonal tonic
● Mild sedative ● Relieves spasm

Menopause Black cohosh has become the herb of choice for treating menopausal symptoms. Although research is divided on its effectiveness, it is well worth trying for relief of menopausal symptoms such as hot flashes, night sweats, disturbed sleep,

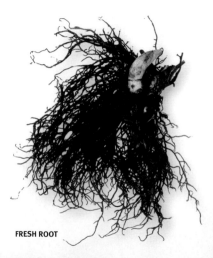

DRIED ROOT

irritability, breast tenderness, menstrual pain, and irregular or absent periods. Again, it may prove more effective in combination with other herbs.

Nerve problems Black cohosh has mild sedative activity and can aid nerve-based problems such as pain, chronic headache, migraine, tinnitus, and vertigo. Traditionally, the herb is seen as a "nervine" (calming and strengthening the nervous system), its overall effect on the nervous system being to reduce overactivity and relieve pain.

KEY INFORMATION

SAFETY	★ ★ ★ ★ ☆
TRADITIONAL USE	★ ★ ★ ★ ★
RESEARCH	★ ★ ★ ☆ ☆

BEST TAKEN AS Tincture ✓✓✓ Capsule ✓✓ Tablet ✓
DOSAGE M, D (*see pp.44–45*)
OFTEN USED WITH Chaste berry (*Vitex agnus-castus*), dong quai (*Angelica sinensis*).
CAUTIONS Do not take during pregnancy and while breast-feeding, except on the advice of an herbal or medical practitioner. Larger doses can cause stomach upsets and headache. Rarely, may cause liver damage; avoid in pre-existing liver disease. See also pp.42–51.

nervous irritability, and headache. It should be taken for at least 2–3 weeks to see if beneficial effects result. It may prove more effective when combined with other suitable herbs like sage (*Salvia officinalis*), particularly when these are recommended by an herbal practitioner. Where nervous exhaustion or depression are present, black cohosh should be combined with St. John's wort (*Hypericum perforatum*). Black cohosh is taken to treat premenstrual problems such as

FRESH ROOT

Arthritis and rheumatism For muscle pain, arthritis, and rheumatic conditions (especially when associated with menopause), black cohosh can sometimes prove highly effective in relieving pain and inflammation and improving freedom of movement. As an antispasmodic, the herb eases cramps and restless muscles, and will tend to help lower raised blood pressure.

Cancer Black cohosh has estrogenic activity within the body, although it appears not to contain estrogens. Opinion varies about the herb's safety in hormone-dependent cancers such as breast and ovarian cancer. In this situation, seek advice from your herbal practitioner or doctor before starting to take black cohosh.

NATIVE AMERICAN REMEDY

The root of black cohosh was commonly used to treat female ailments. Few records show with certainty that black cohosh was widely used by Native American women, but it is known that the root was used to stimulate menstruation, to relieve pain, and to help the flow of breast milk after childbirth.

CHEROKEE WOMAN

Another name for black cohosh is bugbane; its faintly unpleasant smell is said to repel insects.

A remedy for scurvy long before vitamin C was identified, lemon (*Citrus limon*) is a valuable preventative medicine, increasing resistance to infection and helping to maintain good health.

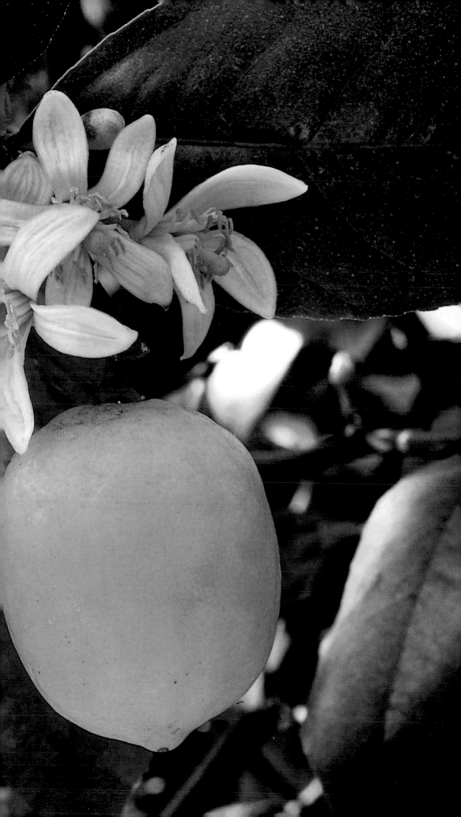

Lemon

Citrus limon

One the most useful home remedies, lemon works well in a host of common complaints. The traditional drink of lemon and honey can be spiced up with ginger and garlic to make a potent brew for colds, flu, coughs, and digestive disorders. Overall, the fruit improves resistance to infection.

MEDICINAL USES

Parts used Essential oil ● Fruit/juice ● Peel ● Seed

Key actions Antioxidant ● Antiseptic ● Detoxifying agent ● Nutritive

Detoxification Most parts of the lemon can be used medicinally. The juice is taken as a cleansing drink, rich in vitamin C and antioxidant bioflavonoids, stimulates liver metabolism and detoxification. Diluted juice of a freshly squeezed lemon makes an excellent pre-breakfast drink. The juice makes an effective mouthwash and gargle; to achieve best results add a pinch of chili (*Capsicum* spp.) for mouth ulcers, gingivitis, and sore throat. It also stimulates the appetite, aids digestion, and improves absorption of iron. Its action on the liver means that it helps to reduce the tendency toward allergic reaction and promotes the elimination of waste products. Avoid drinking the juice neat, as it is strongly acidic and can dissolve tooth enamel. Brush teeth after drinking lemon juice.

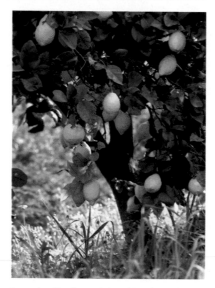

Lemon is said to have originated in India. Its fruit, used as a natural medicine, is harvested in winter when the vitamin C content is at its highest.

juice aids liver metabolism

FRUIT

KEY INFORMATION

SAFETY	★ ★ ★ ★ ★
TRADITIONAL USE	★ ★ ★ ★ ★
RESEARCH	★ ★ ★ ☆ ☆
BEST TAKEN AS	Diluted juice ✓✓✓
DOSAGE	Juice
OFTEN USED WITH	Ginger

(*Zingiber officinalis*)
CAUTIONS Unsuitable in acidic conditions.
See also pp.42–51.

Fungal disorders Lemon seeds, like grapefruit seeds, are antiseptic, and can be taken crushed or chewed to treat candidiasis and other fungal problems. The peel and pith contain high levels of essential oil and bioflavonoids, making extracts valuable supplements for many chronic health problems, including circulatory disorders such as arteriosclerosis, varicose veins, and poor peripheral circulation. Applied topically, the juice and essential oil help to heal acne spots, chilblains, and insect stings and bites. On fungally infected nails, apply 1–2 drops of essential oil a day.

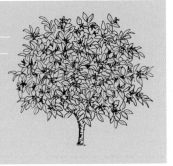

Coffee

Coffea arabica

It is hard to imagine life without coffee culture, but coffee drinking only took off in the West in the 18th century. Coffee's ability to sharpen wit and mental focus, and its effectiveness as a stimulant, has guaranteed its popularity since then.

MEDICINAL USES

Part used Bean (ripe seed)

Key actions Diuretic ● Stimulant

Headache Hard as it may be to think of coffee as a medicine, there is no doubt that it can be put to good medicinal use. Coffee, or caffeine, is a common ingredient in headache and pain-relieving tablets, for example, when used with acetaminophen. On its own, coffee can help to clear a foggy head and headache. In moderation, coffee (and caffeine) stimulates alertness, and improves concentration and work rate.

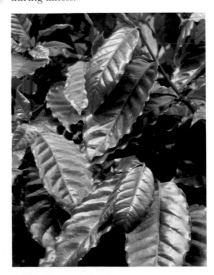

coffee infusion raises level of alertness

COFFEE BEANS

Coffee can, however, cause headache, poor sleep, palpitations, and heart irregularity, although usually only at high levels of intake. Stopping regular coffee intake can lead to headaches lasting for up to 4 days. Its diuretic effect is probably noted by most drinkers. It is best avoided in chronic health problems, especially in long-term weakness and exhaustion.

Forms and flavors Surprisingly, in its percolated form, coffee is the strongest

Coffee originated in Ethiopia. People in the Middle East used it as a religious drink to help them stay awake during prayers.

KEY INFORMATION

SAFETY ★ ★ ★ ★ ☆
TRADITIONAL USE ★ ★ ☆ ☆ ☆
RESEARCH ★ ★ ★ ☆ ☆
BEST TAKEN AS Infusion ✓✓✓
OFTEN USED WITH Cardamom
(*Elettaria cardamomum*)
CAUTIONS Avoid excessive doses, which can cause palpitations.
See also pp.42–51.

(and least healthy); espresso extracts more flavor and less caffeine than other processes. In natural medicine, coffee is thought to put an unnecessary strain on the body, especially during illness.

POWDERED BEANS

Coleus

Coleus forskohlii

In its native India, coleus is used more as a condiment than as a medicine. Its value in health problems such as asthma and high blood pressure has resulted from recent research into the herb's key active constituent, a potent muscle relaxant.

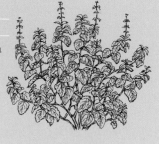

MEDICINAL USES

Parts used Leaf ● Root

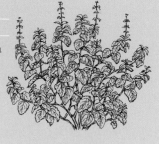

DRIED ROOT

Key actions Antispasmodic ● Dilates blood vessels ● Lowers blood pressure

Cardiovascular problems Coleus, and its key active constituent, forskolin, reduces muscle tension, especially in organs such as the heart and lungs. This antispasmodic action opens up blood vessels, notably the coronary arteries serving the heart, and also relaxes bronchial muscles within the chest. Coleus can therefore prove helpful in conditions such as angina, related heart conditions, and asthma.

Other uses Evidence also suggests that coleus is useful in treating glaucoma, applied locally to the eye.

Coleus leaves have a distinctive scent similar to camphor.

KEY INFORMATION

SAFETY	★ ★ ☆ ☆ ☆
TRADITIONAL USE	★ ☆ ☆ ☆ ☆
RESEARCH	★ ★ ★ ☆ ☆
BEST TAKEN AS	Standardized extract ✓✓✓
DOSAGE	M (*see pp.44–45*)

CAUTIONS Take only on the advice of an herbal or medical practitioner. Interaction with prescribed medicines likely. See also pp.42–51.

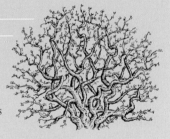

Myrrh

Commiphora molmol

A bitter-tasting resin with an ancient provenance, myrrh has been esteemed as a cleansing and antiseptic remedy for many thousands of years. Used in making perfumes, it powerfully disinfects tissue with which it comes into contact.

MEDICINAL USES

Part used Resin

Key actions Anti-inflammatory
● Antimicrobial ● Antiseptic
● Astringent ● Stimulant

Skin and digestive problems Strongly antiseptic and astringent—and very unpleasant tasting—myrrh is used in inflamed and infected conditions affecting the skin and digestive tract. It makes an excellent mouthwash and gargle, either on its own or combined with other herbs such as sage (*Salvia officinalis*). Diluted (or neat) tincture is a valuable first aid remedy to cleanse and disinfect cuts, scrapes, and wounds; it stings when first being applied, especially the neat tincture.

Cholesterol levels Another antiseptic resin, guggul (*Commiphora mukul*) has a pronounced ability to encourage weight loss and reduce raised cholesterol levels. Research supports its use (in capsule or tablet form) for this purpose.

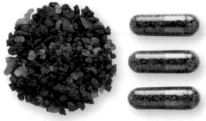

RESIN **CAPSULES**

KEY INFORMATION

SAFETY	★ ★ ★ ⯪ ☆
TRADITIONAL USE	★ ★ ★ ★ ★
RESEARCH	★ ★ ⯪ ☆ ☆

BEST TAKEN AS Diluted tincture (topical) ✓✓✓ Standardized extract: Tablet ✓✓✓ Capsule ✓✓
DOSAGE M (*see pp.44–45*)
CAUTIONS Do not take during pregnancy and while breast-feeding. Can occasionally cause allergy, skin rashes, digestive disturbance, and headache. Avoid taking alcoholic extracts. See also pp.42–51.

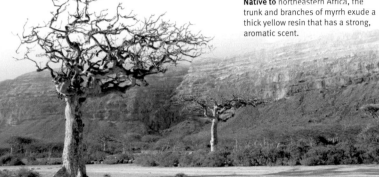

Native to northeastern Africa, the trunk and branches of myrrh exude a thick yellow resin that has a strong, aromatic scent.

Lily of the valley

Convallaria majalis

A slender plant with fragrant white flowers, lily of the valley acts on a weak heart to improve its functioning. A potent medicinal herb, it can have toxic effects.

MEDICINAL USES

Parts used Dried flowering plant • Root

Key actions Diuretic • Heart tonic • Lowers blood pressure

Heart problems The active compounds within lily of the valley are similar to those found in *Digitalis purpurea*, the source of the heart drug *digitoxin*. Lily of the valley is prescribed for functional heart problems since it is milder in action and safer to use.

FLOWERING PLANT

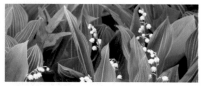

KEY INFORMATION

SAFETY ★ ☆ ☆ ☆ ☆
TRADITIONAL USE ★ ★ ★ ★ ☆
RESEARCH ★ ★ ☆ ☆ ☆
DOSAGE On prescription or in licensed product only.
CAUTIONS Potentially toxic. Do not take if pregnant or breast-feeding. Take only when prescribed by an herbal or medical practitioner. Restricted herb in some countries, including the UK and Australia. See also pp.42–51.

Crataeva, Varuna

Crataeva nurvala

A key remedy for kidney, bladder, and urinary tract problems, crataeva can prove effective in conditions such as cystitis, enlarged prostate, and kidney stones.

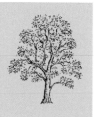

MEDICINAL USES

Parts used Root bark • Stem bark

Key actions Anti-inflammatory • Bladder tonic

Kidney problems Worth considering for any urinary disturbance, crataeva will help to soothe the urinary tract and bladder, reduce frequency, and together with antiseptic remedies, help to clear infections such as cystitis. It is also reputed to help dissolve kidney stones. As are other remedies for the urinary system, crataeva is best taken as a decoction.

KEY INFORMATION

SAFETY ★ ★ ★ ★ ☆
TRADITIONAL USE ★ ★ ★ ★ ☆
RESEARCH ★ ★ ★ ☆ ☆
BEST TAKEN AS Decoction ✓✓✓
Tincture ✓✓
DOSAGE B (*see pp.44–45*)
CAUTIONS Do not take during pregnancy or while breast-feeding. See also pp.42–51.

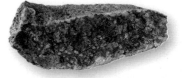

DRIED STEM BARK

Pumpkin seed

Cucurbita pepo

While pumpkins are best known for pie and Halloween, its seeds offer well-established nutritional benefits. Full of high-grade essential fatty acids and trace elements, notably zinc, the seeds make an excellent food supplement.

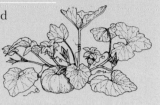

MEDICINAL USES

Parts used Seed ● Seed oil

Key actions Demulcent ● Deworming agent ● Diuretic ● Hormonal agent

Benign prostatic hypertrophy (BPH)
Seeds and seed oil are often used to treat the early stages of enlargement of the prostate gland, or BPH. Recommended by the German Department of Health, the seeds are often effective at relieving BPH symptoms such as difficulty in urination. They do not appear to reverse enlargement of the gland.

Other uses Key constituents within the seeds have an estrogenic activity, so regular intake may prove helpful in relieving menopausal symptoms. The seeds make an effective treatment for worms,

Pumpkin seeds are a good dietary source of iron, zinc, and selenium.

KEY INFORMATION

SAFETY	★ ★ ★ ★ ⯪
TRADITIONAL USE	★ ★ ★ ★ ☆
RESEARCH	★ ★ ★ ⯪ ☆
BEST TAKEN AS	Seed ✓✓✓
DOSAGE	10g a day
OFTEN USED WITH	Saw palmetto (*Serenoa serrulata*)
CAUTIONS	None known. See also pp.42–51.

DRIED SEEDS

seeds are an effective deworming agent

notably tape worm, and can be safely used by children and adults, including during pregnancy. Large quantities need to be taken; seek professional advice.

fruit pulp is used as poultice for burns

Hawthorn

Crataegus spp.

Regarded by herbalists as a "food for the heart," hawthorn is one of the most scientifically validated of all herbal medicines, exerting specific benefit on the heart. Both berries and flowering tops improve blood flow through the coronary arteries to the heart.

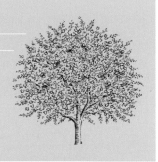

MEDICINAL USES

Parts used Flowering tops ● Fruit ● Leaf

Key actions Antioxidant ● Heart tonic ● Lowers blood pressure ● Relaxes blood vessels

Coronary diseases Hawthorn is not a cure-all for heart and circulatory disorders, but if used carefully and when taken long-term, it will lead to improvement in cardiovascular health. Hawthorn works directly on the heart to slow its rate, improve oxygen uptake, and increase its pumping efficiency. Specific indications include palpitations and heart irregularity, mild angina, and early signs of heart weakness. Evidence from clinical trials supports hawthorn's use in the early stages of heart disease. In such situations, and especially where prescribed medicines are being taken, seek

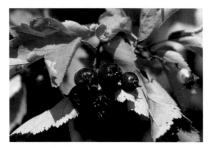

Bright red berries appear in autumn. Although sour in taste, hawthorn berries, like several other red berries, were formerly used to make desserts.

professional advice from an herbal or medical practitioner before starting treatment with the herb.

High and low blood pressure The berries, flowers, and leaves contain high levels of procyanidins, flavonoid compounds which have a strong antioxidant activity that supports healthy circulation. Until recently, the berries were

— berries are used to improve cardiovascular health

DRIED BERRIES

"HEART" OF THE MATTER

In the 19th century, an Irish physician named Dr Green became famous for his secret remedy for heart disease. After his death, it was revealed that his "cure" was actually a tincture made of hawthorn berries.

19TH CENTURY PHYSICIAN

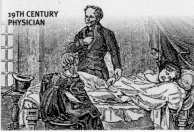

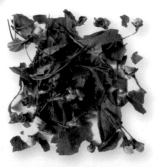

DRIED FLOWERING TOPS

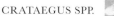
preferred for treating high blood pressure, but the leaves and flowering tops have been shown to have the greatest concentration of procyanidins and are now more commonly used to treat high blood pressure. It is thought that the leaves help to normalize blood pressure by slowing the heart rate and lowering blood pressure in overactive states, and stimulating the heart rate and raising blood pressure in underactive states.

Circulation Hawthorn contains several substances that actively support the health of the arteries, and may also be used to treat or prevent circulatory problems such as atherosclerosis and poor peripheral circulation. Other conditions that may benefit from the herb include intermittent claudication and Raynaud's phenomenon (poor circulation to hands and feet).

KEY INFORMATION

SAFETY	★ ★ ★ ★ ☆
TRADITIONAL USE	★ ★ ★ ★ ☆
RESEARCH	★ ★ ★ ★ ☆

BEST TAKEN AS Standardized extract: Tincture ✓✓✓ Tablet ✓✓ Capsule ✓
DOSAGE M, C (see pp.44–45)
Berry: Not less than 4mg/ml of procyanidins
Leaf: Not less than 10mg/ml of procyanidins
OFTEN USED WITH Yarrow
(Achillea millefolium)
CAUTIONS Interaction with prescribed medicines can occur. Seek advice from an herbal or medical practitioner if taking prescribed medicines, especially for high blood pressure and heart disorders. Rarely, can cause mild symptoms such as headache and digestive upset. See also pp.42–51.

Hawthorn flowers, or May blossoms, were traditionally used in May Day celebrations throughout Europe and have a long association with fertility.

Turmeric

Curcuma longa

A key component of curry mixtures, turmeric's golden-yellow color is familiar to all who eat Indian food. Turmeric root has traditionally been taken to heal allergic and inflammatory conditions and research has established that it has extensive health benefits, due in particular to its strong antioxidant activity.

MEDICINAL USES

Part used Root

Key actions Anti-inflammatory
● Antioxidant ● Protects liver
● Stimulates bile flow

Detoxicant Turmeric promotes healthy function within the upper digestive system as a whole, countering infection and inflammation within the stomach and small intestine. At the same time, it acts to protect the liver from toxic damage and stimulates bile flow.

Cancer prevention Turmeric has a role to play in many chronic health problems and is increasingly being used as a cancer preventative. More controversially, turmeric may be a valuable supplement to take in order to support good health where cancer has been diagnosed. In this case, take the herb only on the recommendation of a qualified herbal practitioner or doctor.

Other uses The root's marked antioxidant activity means that it has a role to play in many chronic illnesses. Recent research suggests possible benefit in conditions as diverse as indigestion and nausea, gastritis, peptic ulcer, liver disorders, high blood cholesterol levels, arthritis, and inflammatory autoimmune problems such as rheumatoid arthritis and Crohn's disease. Less well known is that turmeric also has antifungal and antibacterial activity, and can prove helpful in treating candida infection. The root is also known to slow blood clotting.

KEY INFORMATION

SAFETY	★ ★ ★ ★ ☆
TRADITIONAL USE	★ ★ ★ ★ ☆
RESEARCH	★ ★ ★ ★ ☆

BEST TAKEN AS Tablet ✓✓✓ Powder ✓✓
Tincture ✓
DOSAGE B (*see pp.44–45*)
OFTEN USED WITH Ginger
(*Zingiber officinalis*)
CAUTIONS If taking blood-thinning medication or if gallstones are present, take only on the advice of an herbal or medical practitioner. See also pp.42–51.

turmeric is used as a remedy for gastritis

TURMERIC POWDER

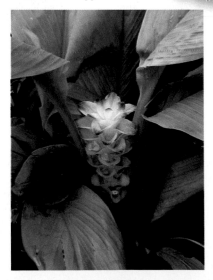

Native to India and southern Asia, turmeric has been used in both Ayurvedic and ancient Chinese herbal medicine to treat liver problems, including jaundice.

Globe artichoke

Cynara scolymus

The flower heads of globe artichoke make a tasty vegetable dish and, like the leaves, have a tonic action on the liver and digestion, stimulating appetite and detoxification. However, the leaves alone are used in medicine, with substantial evidence to prove that they lower cholesterol levels.

MEDICINAL USES

Parts used Flower head (food) • Leaf (medicine)
Key actions Antioxidant • Bitter and digestive tonic • Lowers cholesterol levels • Protects the liver

Liver and kidney problems Another herb where recent research has found new uses, globe artichoke remains a key herb for strengthening liver and kidney function, thus supporting detoxification in chronic conditions such as arthritis, gout, and liver disease.

High cholesterol Clinical trials over the last 30 years have found that globe artichoke leaf lowers cholesterol and triglyceride levels, while high density lipoprotein (HDL) levels tend to increase. The improvement in cholesterol levels varied from 5 to 45 percent, with a daily dose of 7g equivalent of dried leaf. It should be taken for some months to achieve best results. Patients also reported significant relief from symptoms such as nausea, vomiting, abdominal pain, flatulence, and constipation. Following the outcome of these trials, globe artichoke is now commonly taken to treat irritable bowel syndrome and related symptoms such as bloating, abdominal distension, and alternating constipation and diarrhea.

Globe artichoke is a traditional treatment for jaundice and kidney stones.

leaves are used to lower cholesterol levels

DRIED LEAVES

KEY INFORMATION

SAFETY	★ ★ ★ ★ ★
TRADITIONAL USE	★ ★ ★ ★ ☆
RESEARCH	★ ★ ★ ⯪ ☆

BEST TAKEN AS Tablet ✓✓✓ Tincture ✓✓
DOSAGE A (*see pp.44–45*)
OFTEN USED WITH Turmeric (*Curcuma longa*)
CAUTIONS If gallstones are present, take only after consulting an herbal or medical practitioner. Rarely, can cause allergic reactions and gas and bloating. See also pp.42–51.

Native to the Mediterranean, globe artichoke (*Cynara scolymus*) is used both as food and medicine. Its strongly antioxidant and liver-protective leaves are particularly effective.

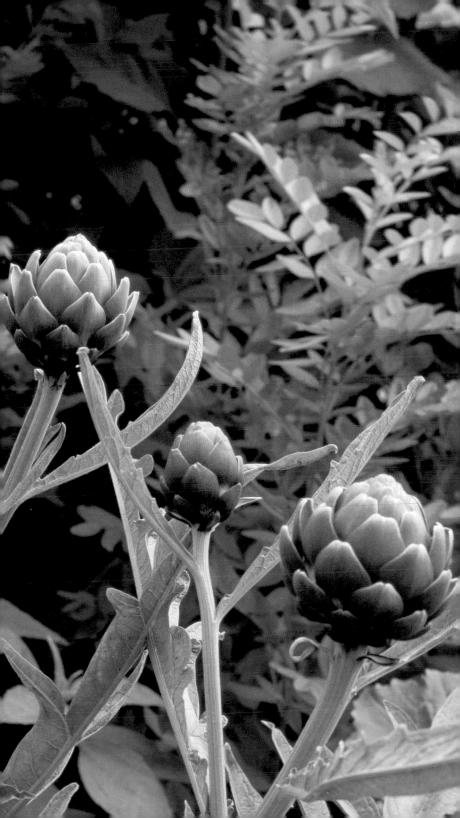

Wild yam

Dioscorea villosa

Increasingly taken as a remedy to relieve menopausal symptoms, wild yam has traditionally been used to ease cramps and muscle pain, especially menstrual pain and colic, throughout the body. A further key use has been in the treatment of inflammatory arthritis, including rheumatoid arthritis.

MEDICINAL USES

Part used Root

Key actions Anti-inflammatory ● Estrogenic ● Relieves spasms

Cramps and pains Wild yam can bring relief wherever cramping pain or over-tensed muscles are the main symptoms. In such a situation, wild yam's combination of antispasmodic and anti-inflammatory activity can help soothe problems as diverse as intestinal cramps, gall bladder pain, menstrual and ovarian pain, and muscle spasm resulting from chronic inflammation. In many cases, the best results will be obtained by combining wild yam with other anti-inflammatory or muscle-relaxant remedies, particularly cramp bark (*Viburnum opulus*). In both osteoarthritis and rheumatoid arthritis, wild yam combines effectively with anti-inflammatories such as devil's claw (*Harpagophytum procumbens*) and willow bark (*Salix alba*).

Menopausal symptoms Wild yam is best known, and most commonly taken, for the relief of menopausal symptoms. Given the herb's undoubted hormonal activity, there

TINCTURE

are good reasons for thinking that it can be taken to improve symptoms such as hot flashes, night sweats, and poor sleep, although it is probable that the steroid compounds in wild yam are not converted to the active hormones in the human body that would thus make it effective for menopausal symptoms; perhaps there is another mechanism at work. Most experts recommend that for best results, the extract should be taken for several weeks to see if it alleviates

KEY INFORMATION

SAFETY	★ ★ ★ ★ ✭
TRADITIONAL USE	★ ★ ★ ✭ ☆
RESEARCH	★ ★ ☆ ☆ ☆

BEST TAKEN AS Tincture ✓✓✓ Capsule ✓✓ Tablet ✓

DOSAGE B (*see pp.44–45*)

OFTEN USED WITH Black cohosh (*Cimicifuga racemosa*)

CAUTIONS Can cause irritation within the digestive tract, usually only with excessive dosage. See also pp.42–51.

tuber contains dioscin

DRIED ROOT

FRESH ROOT

CHOPPED ROOT AND TUBER

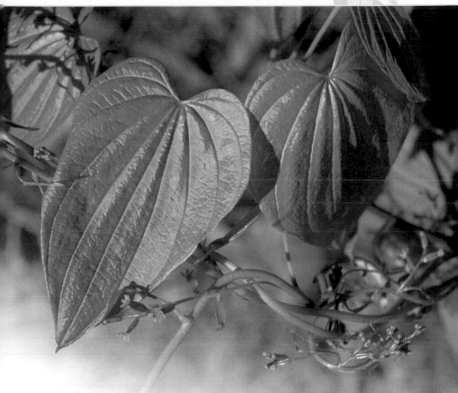

Native to the southern US, Mexico, and Central America, wild yam was known as colic root and rheumatism root, indicating its use by early settlers.

symptoms. Wild yam combines well with black cohosh (*Cimifuga racemosa*) for menopausal and rheumatic problems.

Natural progesterone cream Wild yam natural progesterone cream, applied to the skin rather than taken internally, has received much publicity as a treatment for menopausal problems. A number of clinical studies have failed to find any benefit in relieving symptoms in menopausal women, although there are undoubtedly women who have experienced relief of symptoms with the cream. It is perhaps misleading to describe the product as "natural," as several laboratory processes are required in order to convert the steroidal compounds present in wild yam into progesterone. No plant has yet been found that contains progesterone. That being said, it is the case that hormones processed from natural sources are more readily used by the body than those that are produced synthetically.

Other uses Wild yam has been used within Native American traditions to help prevent miscarriage in the later stages of pregnancy and to relieve pain during childbirth. In keeping with its traditional name of colic root, wild yam makes a useful treatment for irritable bowel and diverticulitis, especially if combined with slippery elm (*Ulmus fulva*).

HORMONES FROM WILD YAM

Wild (and other) yams contain high levels of steroidal compounds, including dioscin, that have an oestrogenic activity. It was the original plant source of diosgenin produced by Japanese scientists in 1936. Diosgenin was synthesized in the laboratory into steroid hormones, and eventually led to the creation of the birth control pill.

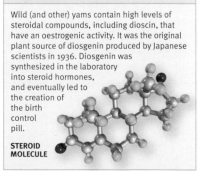

STEROID MOLECULE

Echinacea

Echinacea angustifolia, E. purpurea, E. pallida

A plant from the plains of North America, echinacea is thought to powerfully stimulate the body's ability to resist infection and counter toxicity. Taken mainly as a treatment or preventative for common cold, flu, and viral infections, the herb also helps heal skin disorders such as eczema and acne.

MEDICINAL USES

Parts used Whole plant

Key actions Antibacterial ● Antiviral ● Blood cleanser ● Immune-enhancing ● Wound healer

Colds, flu, viral and bacterial infection
Echinacea—as tincture, tablet, or capsule—is frequently taken to speed recovery from colds, sore throats, and chest infections. The herb is also known to enhance immune resistance in those prone to recurrent colds or herpes outbreaks or where flulike symptoms linger. Echinacea combines well with the flower or berry of elder (*Sambucus nigra*) in this context. The diluted tincture makes a mouthwash or gargle, and can be used to wash infected skin rashes and wounds. Bacterial infections, such as sinusitis, tonsillitis, and chronic bronchitis can be

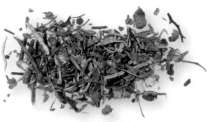

DRIED ROOT

root is used to boost immune system

FRESH ROOT

self-treated with echinacea, preferably in combination with remedies such as garlic (*Allium sativum*) and golden seal (*Hydrastis canadensis*), but a fever of 102°F (39°C) or over indicates the need to seek professional advice. Although the evidence is reasonably good, there is still some debate on echinacea's effectiveness in treating and preventing infection. This may be partly because the dosage used in some clinical trials was too low, or the wrong plant parts or species were studied. The quality and form of echinacea products are

KEY INFORMATION

SAFETY   ★★★★☆
TRADITIONAL USE   ★★★★★
RESEARCH   ★★★☆☆
BEST TAKEN AS Tincture ✓✓✓ Tablet ✓✓ Capsule ✓
DOSAGE B *(see pp.44–45)*
OFTEN USED WITH Golden seal (*Hydrastis canadensis*)
CAUTIONS Can cause allergic reactions. If taking prescribed medication, seek advice from an herbal or medical practitioner. See also pp.41–52.

important—*E. angustifolia* or extracts of the fresh-pressed juice of the above-ground parts of *E. purpurea* are thought to have the strongest medicinal activity.

Immune support and detoxification

Echinacea stimulates nonspecific immunity, increasing the number and activity of white blood cells. This makes it a frontline remedy wherever the immune system is overburdened by chronic infection or toxic residues, such as swollen lymph glands, recurrent boils, chronic dull headache, or sore throat. Used carefully—and this means in conjunction with an herbal practitioner—it helps in cleansing the lymph system, supporting resistance to underlying infection such as fungal problems, and improving overall vitality. Echinacea is not suitable for self-treatment in autoimmune disorders or HIV infection.

SNAKE ROOT

Knowledge of echinacea's medicinal value has been passed down from the experience of Native Americans. Used traditionally as a treatment for snake bite (hence its other common name, "snake root"), echinacea has been used to prevent septic infection in wounds and as a remedy for toothache, sore throat, and rabies.

RATTLESNAKE

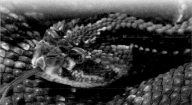

Three echinacea species are used medicinally. All are threatened in the wild, but *Echinacea purpurea* is cultivated widely in the US and Europe.

aerial parts are used to aid recovery from colds and flu

A Native American remedy for septic conditions and snake bites, echinacea (*Echinacea* spp.) is today the most important immune stimulant in Western herbal medicine.

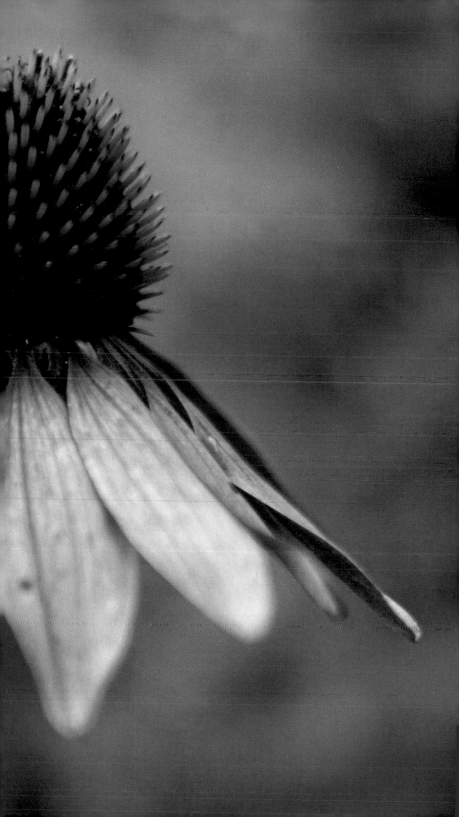

Cardamom

Elettaria cardamomum

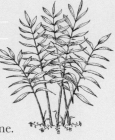

A well-known Indian condiment, cardamom has a warm, slightly spicy taste, and can be added to sweet and savory dishes alike. Its seeds combine well with other remedies to improve flavor and to soothe an upset digestive system. They also add zest to coffee, making a subtler stimulant than coffee alone.

MEDICINAL USES

Parts used Essential ● oil Seed

Key actions Mild stimulant ● Relieves gas ● Soothes digestion ● Tonic

Gas, bloating, digestive ill health

Cardamom's main therapeutic use lies in easing discomfort within the upper digestive system, making it a valuable digestive remedy. Mildly warming and analgesic, its oil relieves colic and gas, and helps settle nausea, griping, and indigestion. It combines well with chamomile (*Chamomilla recutita*). Use crushed seed or tincture; take the essential oil internally only on professional advice.

KEY INFORMATION

SAFETY	★ ★ ★ ★ ★
TRADITIONAL USE	★ ★ ★ ✭ ☆
RESEARCH	★ ★ ✭ ☆ ☆

BEST TAKEN AS Crushed seed ✓✓✓
Tincture ✓✓
DOSAGE C (*see pp.44–45*)
OFTEN USED WITH Ginger (*Zingiber officinalis*)
CAUTIONS None known. See also pp.42–51.

seeds are an effective remedy for bad breath ——

SEEDPODS

Throat and chest problems
The seeds' warming and slightly antiseptic action extends to the throat and chest, making it a good addition to gargles for sore throat, and in chest problems such as asthma and bronchitis.

Male tonic
The long-standing reputation of cardamom as an aphrodisiac, particularly in the Middle East, is supported by the presence of androgenic compounds within the seeds. Cardamom is most likely to be beneficial when combined with herbs such as damiana (*Turnera diffusa*) and Korean ginseng (*Panax ginseng*).

TINCTURE

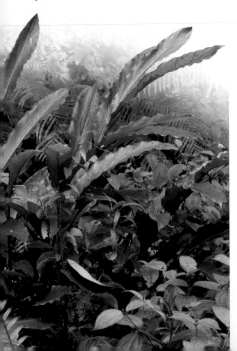

An aromatic herb, cardamom is one of the oldest spices in the world. Apart from its medicinal value, it was also used in perfumes by the ancient Egyptians.

Clove

Eugenia caryophylatta syn. *Syzygium aromaticum*

Originally from the Spice Islands of Indonesia, cloves hold a revered place in oriental herbal medicine and cuisine. A potent antiseptic, cloves added to food help prevent foodborne infection and food poisoning. The essential oil is an excellent first aid remedy for mouth ulcers, toothache, and nerve pain in general.

MEDICINAL USES

Parts used Essential oil
- Flower bud (clove)

Key actions Analgesic • Anti-emetic • Antioxidant • Antiseptic • Astringent • Stimulant

Toothache and nerve pain A clove tucked in the mouth, or one drop of essential oil placed on a cotton ball and plugged into a tooth, is a tried and trusted remedy for toothache. It should be used sparingly and the oil should not be placed on the gum. The diluted oil (maximum 3 percent concentration) may also be applied to the skin to relieve nerve pain elsewhere in the body, such as in shingles.

Digestive upset and irritable bowel syndrome With a positive action on the stomach, small doses of clove powder or tincture make a useful remedy in conditions such as nausea, indigestion, gas, and bloating. Cloves can bring relief in gastroenteritis and diarrhea and can counter infection. Mildly anaesthetic, it is worth trying in irritable bowel syndrome, where it may reduce nerve sensitivity within the gut, easing spasms and urgency.

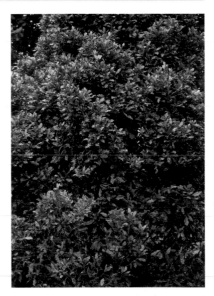

Grown extensively in Tanzania and Madagascar, cloves are originally from the Molucca Islands in Indonesia and the southern Philippines.

oil is extracted from the flowers

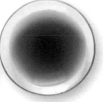

DRIED FLOWER BUDS (CLOVES)

KEY INFORMATION

SAFETY	★★★☆☆
TRADITIONAL USE	★★★★★
RESEARCH	★★★★☆

BEST TAKEN AS Dried flower bud ✓✓✓ Essential oil ✓✓ Tincture ✓
DOSAGE C (*see pp.44–45*)
OFTEN USED WITH Licorice (*Glycyrrhiza glabra*)
CAUTIONS External use can cause dermatitis. Do not take essential oil internally. See also pp.42–51.

FRESH FLOWER BUDS

TINCTURE

Siberian ginseng

Eleutherococcus senticosus

First brought into prominence in the West by Soviet research, Siberian ginseng has been routinely given to Russian cosmonauts to aid endurance in space. Similar to Korean ginseng, Siberian ginseng improves the ability to adapt to all kinds of stress, physical and mental.

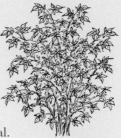

MEDICINAL USES

Part used Root

Key actions Adaptogen • Immune-stimulant • Tonic

Low stamina and endurance Siberian ginseng is a key adaptogen to enhance physical performance and stamina. Research confirms its action in supporting physical endurance and the ability to cope with increased levels of stress and strain, whether these are caused by physical, chemical, environmental, or emotional factors. Its range of indications is therefore very wide, and includes overwork, jetlag, hard physical work, extremes of heat or cold, exposure to radiation, and any situation involving prolonged effort (although not in cases of high blood pressure). For those preparing for exams, Siberian ginseng combines well with

root is taken to improve mental and physical resilience

FRESH ROOT

rosemary (*Rosmarinus officinalis*) and ginkgo (*Ginkgo biloba*). The standard advice is to take the herb for up to 6 weeks at a time, and to avoid caffeine, which is thought to undermine the herb's stamina-building effect.

Tiredness and exhaustion Where vitality is low, Siberian ginseng will usually help to improve energy levels, especially in older adults. Although not all states of tiredness and exhaustion will respond to the herb's tonic qualities, many will, notably where adrenal or thyroid gland function is being compromised by overactivity and lack of opportunity to relax and rest. In severe exhaustion, start with a very low dose and slowly increase. It combines well with golden root (*Rhodiola rosea*) and withania (*Withania somnifera*) where ongoing demands make adequate rest hard to come by.

tincture is taken as a general tonic

TINCTURE

KEY INFORMATION

SAFETY   ★ ★ ★ ★ ☆
TRADITIONAL USE ★ ★ ★ ★ ☆
RESEARCH   ★ ★ ★ ☆ ☆
BEST TAKEN AS Standardized extract: Tincture ✓✓✓ Tablet ✓✓
DOSAGE C (see pp.44–45)
CAUTIONS Not advisable in high blood pressure. May interact with other medication. See also pp.42–51.

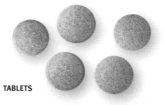

TABLETS

Similar in many ways to Korean ginseng (*Panax ginseng*), Siberian ginseng helps to maintain performance and a sense of well-being when one is under long-term stress.

Chronic illness

Siberian ginseng can provide much-needed support in times of poor health. Usually in combination with other immune-stimulant remedies, its immune-enhancing and tonic properties make it suitable for chronic viral infections such as shingles, glandular fever, and chronic fatigue syndrome. Even in severe illness, Siberian ginseng can contribute to an improved quality of life, and can be considered specifically for convalescence. In debilitated states and convalescence, Siberian ginseng is best taken for several months at a low to medium dosage. It is most likely to strengthen vitality when any improvement in energy levels is used to nurture a return to good health, and not spent on meeting external demands such as work.

Cancer A valuable remedy to aid recovery after surgery or radiation therapy, it plays a role in supporting people with cancer where immune resistance needs to be strengthened, and the ability to tolerate chemotherapy improved. Professional advice must be sought in such cases, not least because the herb can interact with other medication.

ADAPTOGENS

The term adaptogen was coined by Soviet scientists Lazarev and Brekhman in the 1960s to describe herbal medicines that enabled the body and mind to respond more effectively to stress of all kinds. Following research into Siberian ginseng, Russian cosmonauts have used extracts of the herb as an adaptogen to aid stamina and improve the ability to cope with weightlessness.

COSMONAUT'S MEDAL

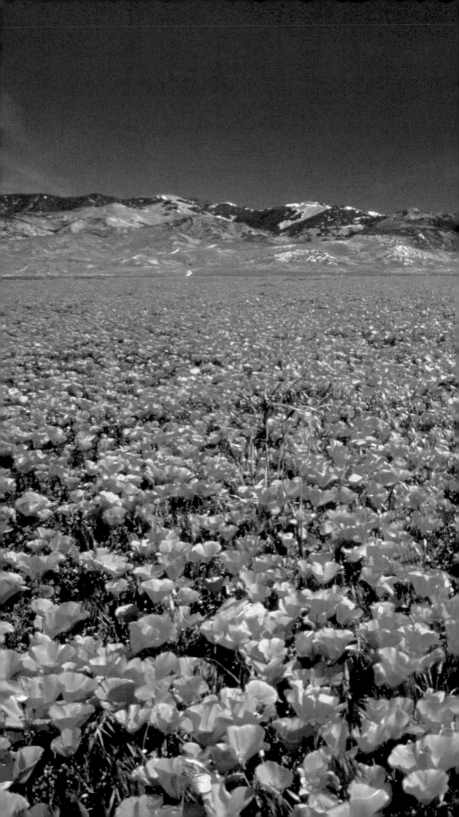

Californian poppy (*Eschscholzia californica*) is a native of grassy areas of western North America. Its gently sedative and analgesic qualities make it a valuable remedy for anxiety and pain.

Californian poppy

Eschscholzia californica

Although a close relative of the opium poppy, Californian poppy is safe and non-addictive, and makes a gentle and effective sedative for children.

MEDICINAL USES

Part used   Aerial parts

Key actions   Mild analgesic ● Mild sedative ● Relaxant

Sleep difficulties   Best taken in the evening for short-term sleep disturbance, Californian poppy improves sleep quality and can be helpful for nightmares and bedwetting. It combines well with passion flower (*Passiflora incarnata*).

FLOWERS

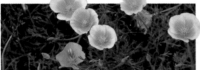

Children's remedy   Californian poppy soothes overactivity and also benefits conditions involving pain or anxiety such as headache, migraine, and irritability.

KEY INFORMATION

SAFETY	★ ★ ★ ★ ☆
TRADITIONAL USE	★ ★ ★ ☆ ☆
RESEARCH	★ ★ ☆ ☆ ☆

DOSAGE   C (*see pp.44–45*)

CAUTIONS   None known within normal dosage, but may have addictive effects with alcohol or other sedative herbs/medication. Long-term use not advised. See also pp.42–51.

Eucalyptus

Eucalyptus globulus

A key aboriginal remedy of Australia, eucalyptus can be used to treat everything from colds and chest infection to skin conditions and fever.

MEDICINAL USES

Parts used   Essential oil ● Leaf

KEY INFORMATION

SAFETY	★ ★ ★ ★ ☆
TRADITIONAL USE	★ ★ ★ ★ ★
RESEARCH	★ ★ ★ ★ ☆

BEST TAKEN AS   Manufactured products ✓✓✓

DOSAGE   M (*see pp.44–45*)

CAUTIONS   Not suitable for children under 5. Do not take essential oil internally, except on professional advice. Overuse of the oil topically may be dangerous. See also pp.42–51.

Key actions   Antiseptic ● Expectorant

Coughs and colds   The oil is used in many over-the-counter preparations. Main uses include cold symptoms with or without feverishness, nasal and sinus congestion, sore throat, and phlegmy cough.

Skin problems

Apply an infusion of the leaves or diluted oil (maximum 5 percent concentration) to insect bites and fungal skin conditions.

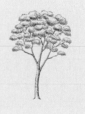

FLOWERING STEM

Eyebright

Euphrasia officinalis

Eyebright may have gained its name from its flowers, thought to resemble the human eye. More probably, experience taught that the herb was good for the eyes, hence the name. Although little researched, it contains constituents known to have a tonic effect on mucous membranes, including those of the eyes.

MEDICINAL USES

Part used Whole herb

Key actions Anti-catarrhal ● Anti-inflammatory ● Astringent

Eye disorders In Western herbal medicine, eyebright is a specific remedy for common eye problems such as conjunctivitis ("red eye") and blepharitis (infection of the eyelid). Taken internally, it is thought to heal the surface of the eye, relieving inflammation and drying up excessive watering. Well-filtered, cooled eyebright infusion can also be applied as a lotion to a partially closed eye. Traditionally, the herb has been taken to improve vision.

leaves are used to relieve inflammation of the eye

DRIED LEAVES

Catarrh and hay fever Routinely taken by hay fever sufferers each summer, eyebright helps to control allergic symptoms such as sneezing, itchy eyes, and copious watery mucus. Similar conditions that affect the ear, nose, and throat are also likely to benefit from its use.

KEY INFORMATION

SAFETY   ★ ★ ★ ★ ☆
TRADITIONAL USE   ★ ★ ★ ★ ☆
RESEARCH   ★ ★ ☆ ☆ ☆
BEST TAKEN AS Infusion ✓✓✓
Tincture ✓✓ Tablet, capsule ✓
DOSAGE B (*see pp.44–45*)
OFTEN USED WITH Elder (*Sambucus nigra*)
CAUTIONS Possible eye irritation when used topically. See also pp.42–51.

Poorly researched, eyebright is regarded by herbalists as a key remedy for mucous membranes of the eyes, ears, and sinuses.

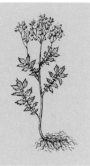

Meadowsweet

Filipendula ulmaria

Aspirin-like substances were first isolated in the 19th century from meadowsweet. The herb has some of the characteristic properties of aspirin, notably a mild anti-inflammatory activity, but unlike aspirin, meadowsweet is a key remedy for healing acid-related problems such as heartburn and gastric ulcer.

MEDICINAL USES

Part used Flowering top

Key actions Antacid ● Anti-inflammatory ● Antirheumatic ● Astringent

Acid indigestion, gastric ulcer, irritable bowel One of the best remedies for acidic digestive problems, meadowsweet promotes stomach repair while controlling acid release. Taken symptomatically, meadowsweet tea relieves mild heartburn or acid reflux, although for best results, meadowsweet may need to be taken long-term. The herb's astringent, binding quality makes it a useful treatment for chronic diarrhea and irritable bowel.

Native to Europe, meadowsweet flourishes in damp places.

Rheumatic aches and pains, fibromyalgia Meadowsweet can bring relief to stiff, sore, and aching muscles and joints, soothing inflammation and stimulating clearance of acid residues. Where symptoms get worse on waking or sitting for long periods, combine it with celery seed (*Apium graveolens*) in order to ease inflammation and aid free movement.

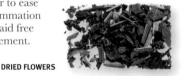

DRIED FLOWERS

KEY INFORMATION

SAFETY	★ ★ ★ ★ ⯪
TRADITIONAL USE	★ ★ ★ ⯪ ☆
RESEARCH	★ ★ ⯪ ☆ ☆

BEST TAKEN AS Infusion ✓✓✓ Tincture ✓✓

DOSAGE A (*see pp.44–45*)

OFTEN USED WITH Celery seed (*Apium graveolens*)

CAUTIONS Contains aspirin-like substances; if allergic to aspirin, do not use. Can cause gastrointestinal upset. See also pp.42–51.

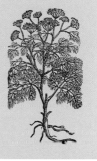

Fennel

Foeniculum vulgare

Fennel tea's pleasant flavor and aroma make it a refreshing drink with marked benefits for digestive health. Safe for children, it gently warms and stimulates appetite and digestion, in the process relieving colic, gas, and bloating. Traditional use is wide-ranging, from relieving menstrual pain to shortness of breath.

MEDICINAL USES

Parts used Seed ● Essential oil

Key actions Eases gas and cough
● Improves appetite and digestion
● Increases breast milk

Indigestion, gas, bloating, colic
Fennel's pleasant taste makes it a popular remedy for upper digestive problems. It relieves griping and abdominal bloating, clears trapped gas, and improves appetite. The diluted tea can be given to young children to relieve colic and teething pain, and is also known to reduce food cravings.

Sore throat, cough, congestion Fennel
tea makes an effective gargle, soothing mucous membranes and relieving cough.

KEY INFORMATION

SAFETY	★ ★ ★ ★ ☆
TRADITIONAL USE	★ ★ ★ ★ ☆
RESEARCH	★ ★ ★ ☆ ☆
BEST TAKEN AS	Infusion ✓✓✓
DOSAGE	C (*see pp.44–45*)

OFTEN USED WITH Peppermint (*Mentha x piperita*)
CAUTION Can cause allergic reaction. Do not exceed recommended dose or take for long periods of time. See also pp.42–51.

DRIED SEEDS

Hormonal benefits
Fennel increases the production of breast milk and may be taken to start or to maintain a sufficient flow of milk. Taken over a few months, fennel can help improve menstrual regularity and will tend to reduce menstrual cramps. The seed has a long-standing reputation as an aid to weight loss and can be added to the diet when trying to lose weight.

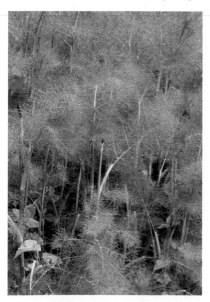

seeds are used to aid digestion

As early as Roman times, fennel was thought to control obesity; a tea made from the seed normalizes the appetite.

FLOWERING HERB

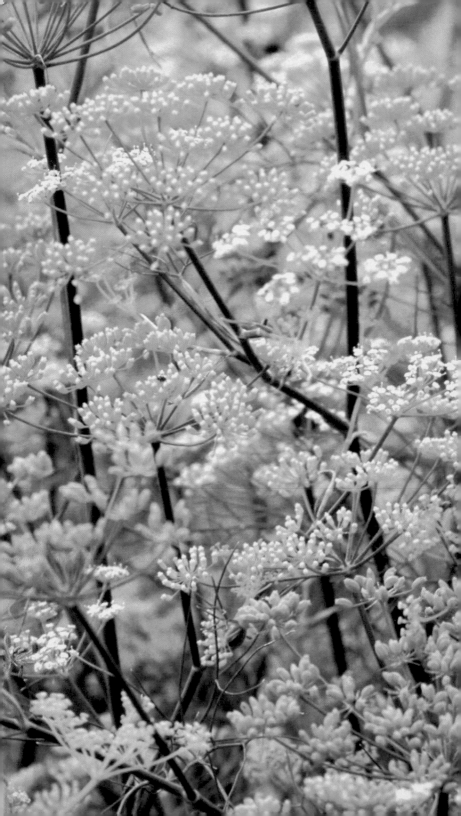

The umbels of golden-yellow flowers and dark green, soft feathery leaves make fennel (*Foeniculum vulgare*) easily recognizable in the pastures and gardens where it grows.

Bladderwrack, Kelp

Fucus vesiculosis

A cool-water sea vegetable, bladderwrack absorbs large quantities of minerals from the sea. Containing significant levels of iodine—the mineral most responsible for stimulating thyroid gland function—bladderwrack has traditionally been used as part of a weight-loss regime.

MEDICINAL USES

Part used Plant (thallus)

Key actions Demulcent ● Nutritive ● Stimulates thyroid gland ● Supports weight loss

Weight loss and underactive thyroid gland Although as yet unconfirmed by research, anecdotal evidence suggests that bladderwrack is an effective supplement in weight-loss regimes where the thyroid gland is underactive. The herb is a specific used for low thyroid function—a condition that causes low vitality, depressed mood and mental function, weight gain, and sensitivity to cold. It can quickly help to reverse symptoms where the thyroid gland is only mildly underactive, or where iodine deficiency is the principal problem. Treating thyroid disorders can be very complicated and it is advisable to seek professional advice for an apparently underactive thyroid.

Other uses Containing minerals that include iodine, silicon, zinc, and copper, bladderwrack is linked to low thyroid

KEY INFORMATION

SAFETY	★ ★ ★ ★ ☆
TRADITIONAL USE	★ ★ ★ ★ ☆
RESEARCH	★ ★ ⯪ ☆ ☆
BEST TAKEN AS	Capsule, tablet ✓✓✓
DOSAGE	B (*see pp.44–45*)

CAUTIONS Do not take during pregnancy, while breast-feeding, or when thyroid is overactive. See also pp.42–51.

function or mineral deficiency. Bladderwrack also supports the elasticity and overall health of arteries. With a none-too-pleasant taste, it is best taken in capsule or tablet form. It will improve arthritic and rheumatic symptoms where these are linked to low thyroid function. While it is safe at normal dosage, bladderwrack can have adverse effects on the thyroid gland. It can also be contaminated by heavy metals, so quality control is essential.

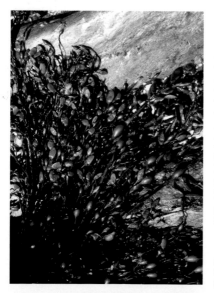

seaweed extracts can aid weight loss

DRIED SEAWEED

Native to North Atlantic shores and the western Mediterranean sea, bladderwrack is a brownish-green sea plant rich in iodine and silicon.

Reishi, Ling-zhi

Ganoderma lucidum

Used for over 4,000 years in China, Japan, and Korea, reishi mushroom has traditionally been taken as a calming tonic in old age. It has also been used for many age-related health problems, including heart and liver disease, inflammatory arthritis, and cancer.

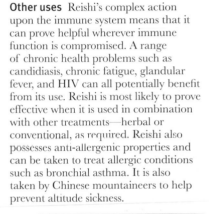

MEDICINAL USES

Part used Fungus

Key actions Antioxidant ● Anticancer ● Heart tonic ● Protects liver

Anticancer remedy Scientific studies are beginning to validate some of reishi's traditional uses: extracts have been shown to stimulate immune function and promote antitumor activity. A safe remedy, reishi is increasingly being used as a supplementary treatment in cancer, especially during chemotherapy. In this situation, reishi supports both immune and liver function. In cancer and other serious illnesses, take only on professional advice. While it is thought to have low toxicity, long-term use (more than three months) may cause side effects.

Other uses Reishi's complex action upon the immune system means that it can prove helpful wherever immune function is compromised. A range of chronic health problems such as candidiasis, chronic fatigue, glandular fever, and HIV can all potentially benefit from its use. Reishi is most likely to prove effective when it is used in combination with other treatments—herbal or conventional, as required. Reishi also possesses anti-allergenic properties and can be taken to treat allergic conditions such as bronchial asthma. It is also taken by Chinese mountaineers to help prevent altitude sickness.

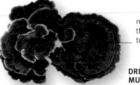

reishi protects the liver from toxic damage

DRIED MUSHROOMS

Found growing wild on tree trunks or stumps in coastal China, reishi mushrooms are now widely cultivated in North America, Japan, and Korea.

KEY INFORMATION

SAFETY	★★★★✬
TRADITIONAL USE	★★★★☆
RESEARCH	★★★☆☆

BEST TAKEN AS Standardized extract ✓✓✓ Tincture ✓✓

DOSAGE M (*see pp.44–45*)

OFTEN USED WITH Shiitake (*Lentinus edodes*)

CAUTIONS Can cause allergic reactions. See also pp.42–51.

Gentian

Gentiana lutea

Containing some of the most bitter-tasting substances on the planet, gentian is classified in herbal medicine as a "pure" bitter.

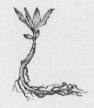

MEDICINAL USES

Part used Root

Key actions Bitter • Digestive tonic

Weak digestion Like all bitters, gentian works to stimulate and strengthen digestive activity. A few drops of gentian tincture is best used for weak digestion in elderly people and convalescing patients. It stimulates liver and pancreatic function and the release of stomach acid. Increased digestive juices also lead to a healthier appetite.

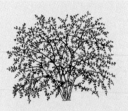

FLOWERS

root stimulates digestion

DRIED ROOT

KEY INFORMATION

SAFETY	★★★★☆
TRADITIONAL USE	★★★★★
RESEARCH	★★★★☆
BEST TAKEN AS	Tincture ✓✓✓
DOSAGE	D (*see pp.44–45*)
CAUTIONS	None known. See also pp. 42–51.

Gymnema, Gurmar

Gymnema sylvestris

Long used in India to treat diabetes and poor sugar tolerance, gymnema stimulates insulin production and may help pancreatic function.

MEDICINAL USES

Part used Leaf

Key actions Antidiabetic • Lowers blood sugar levels

Sugar craving and poor sugar tolerance
Gymnema's traditional name of "gurmar" means "sugar destroyer," gained because it neutralizes the sweet tastebuds in the tongue and tackles sugar cravings. Take 20–50 drops of tincture on the tongue every 3 hours. Larger doses are required to improve prediabetic states and diabetes, which should be treated only on the advice of a health professional.

KEY INFORMATION

SAFETY	★★★★☆
TRADITIONAL USE	★★★★☆
RESEARCH	★★★☆☆
BEST TAKEN AS	Tincture ✓✓✓
DOSAGE	D (*see pp.44–45*)
CAUTIONS	Will interact with conventional medication for diabetes. See also pp.42–51.

LEAVES

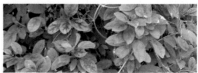

Soy

Glycine max

Most familiar as soy sauce or tofu, soy appears to confer significant health benefits if used regularly. As food, soy is rich in protein, lecithin, and essential fatty acids; as medicine, it contains isoflavones and other compounds, which have estrogenic and antioxidant activity.

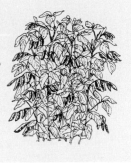

MEDICINAL USES

Parts used Bean ● Sprout

Key actions Estrogenic ● Nutritive

Menopausal problems Several clinical trials have showed that concentrated soy extracts help relieve menopausal problems such as hot flashes. These phytoestrogen-rich extracts are an option when considering natural alternatives for menopause, but are best taken only where other approaches have failed to work. Soy sprouts, beans, and fermented products—as part of a balanced diet—provide a good input of nutrients and phytoestrogens, especially during menopause. Sprouts are preferable to beans, since they are more nutritious, richer in phytoestrogens, and, unlike beans, do not impair absorption of vitamins and minerals, notably iron.

Raised cholesterol levels Soy lecithin is a useful supplement, with research endorsing its ability to lower raised cholesterol levels.

KEY INFORMATION

SAFETY ★★★★☆
TRADITIONAL USE ★★★☆☆
RESEARCH ★★★☆☆
BEST TAKEN AS Sprouts ✓✓✓
DOSAGE Food, M (*see pp.44–45*)
OFTEN USED WITH Black cohosh (*Cimicifuga racemosa*)
CAUTIONS Beans and sprouts can cause allergy. Concentrated extracts may be unsafe for long periods of time due to concerns about estrogenic effects and connections to cancer. Occasionally can cause gastrointestinal upset. See also pp.42–51.

SOY BEANS

SEEDPODS

A staple food in much of Asia, soy has been used in China for at least 5,000 years. It is today one of the world's most important food crops.

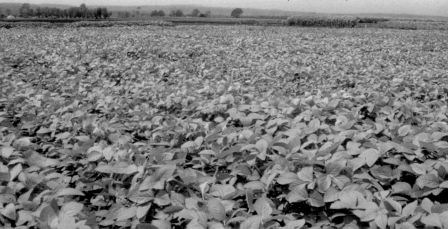

Ginkgo

Ginkgo biloba

Harvested from the world's oldest surviving tree, ginkgo leaf extracts have been shown to markedly improve blood flow through the arteries in the brain, to protect the central nervous system from oxidative damage, and to enhance mental recall and ability in healthy adults.

MEDICINAL USES

Parts used Fruit ● Leaf

Key actions Antioxidant ● Circulatory stimulant ● Improves mental performance ● Protects nerve tissue

Failing memory and mental faculty

Research evidence supports ginkgo's use to strengthen memory and cognitive function. In particular, ginkgo helps to treat and slow down the deterioration in mental function that occurs in dementia and Alzheimer's disease. Well tolerated and rarely causing side effects, ginkgo is a preferred initial treatment for these all too common conditions. Ginkgo can also prove useful in helping control the symptoms of Parkinson's disease. It combines well with golden root (*Rhodiola rosea*).

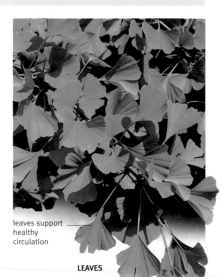

leaves support healthy circulation

LEAVES

Dizziness and tinnitus By improving blood flow to the central nervous system, ginkgo can benefit nerve-related problems such as dizziness, vertigo, nerve deafness, and tinnitus (ringing in the ears). Although such conditions can be very difficult to treat effectively, ginkgo is well worth trying for possible improvement in symptoms.

KEY INFORMATION

SAFETY	★★★⯪☆
TRADITIONAL USE	★★★★☆
RESEARCH	★★★★★

BEST TAKEN AS Standardized extract: Tablet ✓✓✓ Tincture ✓✓
DOSAGE M (*see pp.44–45*)
CAUTIONS If taking prescribed medication, especially anticoagulant treatment, take only on after consulting an herbal or medical practitioner. Can occasionally cause headache or gastrointestinal upset. See also pp.42–51.

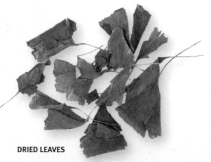

DRIED LEAVES

Poor peripheral circulation Ginkgo stimulates blood flow throughout the body, from the head to the hands and feet. It can help with weak circulation, including altitude sickness, low blood pressure, Raynaud's syndrome, and intermittent claudication.

BEYOND THE GREAT WALL

Once thought by Western scientists to be extinct, ginkgoes were rediscovered in Japan in 1691. They had spread by seed from China, where they were mainly found in Buddhist monasteries, cultivated since c.1100 CE for medicinal uses.

PAGODA

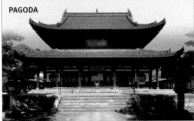

Ginkgo trees are widely cultivated in China, France, and the USA.

leaves help to stabilize nerve function

Other uses Given ginkgo's positive action on the circulation and central nervous system, it would be surprising if there weren't further indications for its use. In particular, ginkgo is taken on a daily basis by people aged 50 and over to support healthy circulation and mental function. As well as protecting nerve tissue from damage, it helps to ensure an adequate blood supply to the central nervous system. With professional advice, ginkgo can also be taken for conditions as varied as asthma, depression, frost bite, glaucoma, and multiple sclerosis.

Licorice

Glycyrrhiza glabra

Tonic and anti-inflammatory, this most versatile of herbs finds use in treating ill health of all kinds. Added routinely to herbal prescriptions, licorice acts on the adrenal glands and seems to reinforce the action and improve the flavor of herbs with which it is combined.

MEDICINAL USES

Part used Root

Key actions Anti-inflammatory
● Antiviral ● Demulcent
● Expectorant ● Tonic

Gastritis, peptic ulcer, inflammatory bowel disease Licorice's soothing, healing action works throughout the gastrointestinal tract, making it applicable in any situation where the gut or stomach wall is inflamed or ulcerated. Licorice tea taken at night can help ease acid reflux.

Inflammatory arthritis Licorice's anti-inflammatory action serves to relieve stiffness, heat, and pain in muscles and joints.
Working in a manner not too dissimilar to prescribed steroids, it helps to dampen chronic inflammation, easing associated discomfort in conditions such as rheumatoid arthritis and polymyalgia rheumatica.

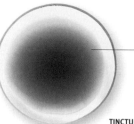

tincture is useful in many inflammatory conditions

TINCTURE

Mouth ulcers, sore throat, bronchitis, cough On its own or in combination with other herbs, licorice tea makes an effective, pleasant-tasting mouthwash or gargle for sore tongue, mouth and throat ulcers, and laryngitis. Swallowed, its demulcent action soothes irritation and inflammation within the airways, such as in bronchial infection, helping to ease cough and stimulate the clearance of phlegm. The herb also appears to protect against tooth decay.

Viral infections Not really an herb to use on its own in this context, licorice combines well with other immune-enhancing herbs to strengthen the body's capacity to counter viral (and

KEY INFORMATION

SAFETY	★ ★ ★ ½ ☆
TRADITIONAL USE	★ ★ ★ ★ ★
RESEARCH	★ ★ ★ ★ ☆

BEST TAKEN AS Tincture ✓✓✓
Capsule ✓✓ Dried root ✓
DOSAGE C (*see pp.44–45*)
OFTEN USED WITH Echinacea
(*Echinacea purpurea*)
CAUTIONS Do not take large doses if you have high blood pressure. During pregnancy or for long-term use, consult an herbal or medical practitioner before using. See also pp.42–51.

root has tonic properties

FRESH ROOT

DRIED ROOT PIECES

other) infections. Among other conditions, licorice has been recommended for chronic fatigue syndrome, mononucleosis, Lyme disease, shingles, and tonsillitis.

Adrenal tonic Licorice can provide valuable support in any situation where the adrenal glands have been subject to long-term stress. It makes an effective tonic in aiding recovery from illness and chronic exhaustion. An estrogenic remedy, it can be particularly helpful in menopausal exhaustion.

Other uses Research in China indicates that licorice can prove helpful in polycystic ovary syndrome, improving menstrual regularity and fertility. It also supports liver function and soothes mucous membranes in the stomach and airways. Licorice makes a valuable tonic to aid recovery from illness and the return to good health.

SWEET COURAGE

The medicinal value of licorice was championed by the ancient Greek commander Alexander the Great (356–323 BCE). It is said his troops chewed on licorice roots before a battle to give them fighting energy, which would have been derived from its effect on their blood sugar and adrenal glands. Soldiers also used it to quench thirst while marching, and thought it helped them stop shaking with fright during battle.

ALEXANDER THE GREAT

Known as the "sweet herb," licorice contains glycyrrhizic acid, which is 50 times sweeter than sugar.

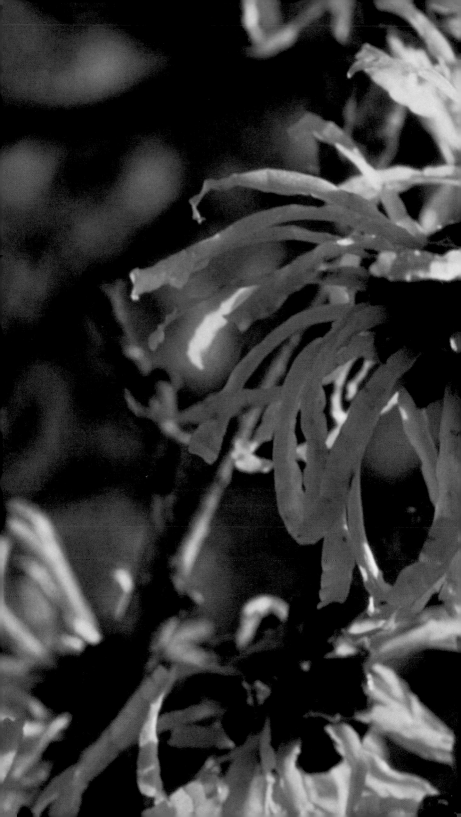

A key astringent remedy for inflamed skin and eye disorders, witch hazel (*Hamamelis virginiana*) was used by early European settlers, who learned its properties from Native American Indians.

Witch hazel

Hamamelis virginiana

Produced by distilling the bark and leaves of this North American tree, witch hazel water is a useful skin cleanser and tonic. A frequent ingredient in cosmetics such as anti-wrinkle creams, the distilled water heals sore, roughened, or inflamed skin.

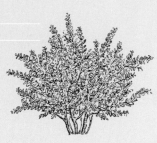

MEDICINAL USES

Parts used Bark ● Leaf

Key actions Anti-inflammatory ● Astringent ● Styptic (stops bleeding)

Eye problems For sore or inflamed eyes, grit, or an insect in the eye, soak cotton wool or lint in witch hazel water and place on the (closed) affected eye. Allow some liquid to enter the eye. For a better effect, add 5–10 drops of witch hazel water and a few grains of salt to an eyebath of clean warm water, and bathe the eye thoroughly, repeating as required.

Bruises, cuts, skin rashes, herpes sores Witch hazel is a useful cleanser for cuts and grazes, stopping blood flow at the same time.

In seeping skin conditions, witch hazel water will help to dry up the leaking fluid and calm irritation. Mildly antiviral, the water can lessen pain in herpes sores.

Varicose veins, capillary fragility, hemorrhoids Witch hazel tones and tightens irritated and over-relaxed tissue. Either witch hazel water or cream makes a first-rate application for varicose veins and hemorrhoids, controlling inflammation and toning distended veins. Thread veins can also benefit.

leaves and twigs are used to make witch hazel water

LEAVES

KEY INFORMATION

SAFETY	★ ★ ★ ★ ★
TRADITIONAL USE	★ ★ ★ ★ ☆
RESEARCH	★ ★ ★ ★ ☆

BEST TAKEN AS Topical: Distilled water or infusion ✓✓✓
DOSAGE T (*see pp.44–45*)
OFTEN USED WITH Aloe vera (*Aloe* spp.)
CAUTION None known. No longer used internally. See also pp.42–51.

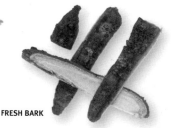

FRESH BARK

A woodland tree native to Canada and eastern parts of the US, witch hazel is today commonly grown for its attractive winter flowers.

Devil's claw

Harpagophytum procumbens

With extensive traditional use for fevers, stomach ache, and rheumatic disease in its native southern Africa, devil's claw is now one of the most scientifically validated herbal medicines for rheumatic and arthritic disorders.

MEDICINAL USES

Part used Secondary root or tuber

Key actions Analgesic ● Anti-inflammatory ● Antirheumatic ● Bitter

Arthritic and rheumatic symptoms

Perhaps the first herbal remedy to be considered for joint and muscle pain, devil's claw can relieve arthritic pain and inflammation, slowing or preventing deterioration in symptoms. Clinical studies have shown devil's claw extracts to be effective in relieving arthritic pain in the knee, hip, and back; patients were also able to reduce their intake of prescribed non-steroidal anti-inflammatories. Osteoarthritis, gout, fibromyalgia, and back pain can all benefit from this herb. Devil's claw is best taken before symptoms demand attention, especially if suitable dietary changes are also made. A distinctly bitter remedy, the tincture will help to stimulate appetite and absorption.

Devil's claw grows in semi-desert conditions and is increasingly rare in the wild. It is now being cultivated organically in Namibia; use organic where possible.

KEY INFORMATION

SAFETY	★★★☆☆
TRADITIONAL USE	★★★★⯪
RESEARCH	★★★★☆

BEST TAKEN AS Standardized extract: Tablet ✓✓✓
DOSAGE M (*see pp.44–45*)
OFTEN USED WITH Willow bark (*Salix alba*)
CAUTIONS With gallstones and peptic ulcer, take only on the advice of an herbal or medical practitioner. Do not take during pregnancy. May cause diarrhea or interact with medications. See also pp.42–51.

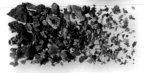

tuber has anti-inflammatory properties

DRIED ROOT

CHOPPED ROOT

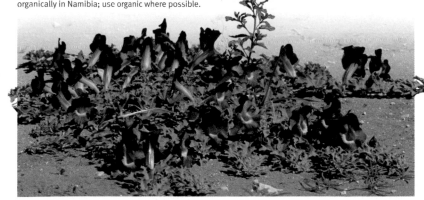

Sea buckthorn

Hippophae rhamnoides

With high levels of minerals and vitamins A and C, sea buckthorn's tart-tasting berries make an ideal supplement to prevent colds and sore throats.

MEDICINAL USES

Part used Flowers ● Fruit ● Leaves ● Seeds

Key actions Antioxidant ● Circulatory tonic ● Rich in vitamins and minerals

Infection As a natural supplement, the juice or syrup of sea buckthorn will improve resistance to colds, sore throat, and sinus problems.

BERRIES

Atherosclerosis, poor circulation to the retina and eye Rich in antioxidant bioflavonoids, sea buckthorn supports capillary and arterial health when taken long-term.

KEY INFORMATION

SAFETY ★★★★★
TRADITIONAL USE ★★★☆☆
RESEARCH ★★★☆☆
BEST TAKEN AS Juice, infusion ✓✓✓
DOSAGE M, C (*see pp.44–45*)
CAUTIONS May increase the risk of bleeding, especially when combined with certain herbs or blood-thinning medications. See also pp.42–51.

Hops

Humulus lupulus

Famed for their bitter taste when used to make beer, hops are a strong sedative and a common ingredient in many over-the-counter sleep remedies.

MEDICINAL USES

Part used Flower (strobile)

Key actions Bitter tonic ● Estrogenic ● Sedative

KEY INFORMATION

SAFETY ★★★½☆
TRADITIONAL USE ★★★★☆
RESEARCH ★★★½☆
BEST TAKEN AS Tincture ✓✓✓ Tablet ✓✓ Capsule ✓
DOSAGE C (*see pp.44–45*)
CAUTIONS Do not take during depression. Can cause drowsiness. See also pp.42–51.

Disturbed sleep To aid sleep, hops are best used in combination with other sedative remedies such as passion flower (*Passiflora incarnata*). Hops' estrogenic action makes them potentially helpful in small doses for menopausal night sweats.

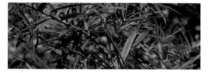

HOP STROBILES

Weak digestion, irritable bowel A few drops of hops tincture taken before meals stimulate appetite. With herbs such as chamomile (*Chamomilla recutita*), hops can help to relieve irritable bowel.

Goldenseal

Hydrastis canadensis

A potent herbal medicine, goldenseal merits its reputation as a remedy that shifts chronic infection and heals weakened and congested mucous membranes. Its key use lies in the treatment of chronic bacterial, fungal, or viral infection affecting mucous membranes anywhere in the body.

MEDICINAL USES

Part used Root

Key actions Anti-inflammatory
● Antimicrobial ● Antibacterial
● Blood cleanser ● Mucous membrane tonic ● Protects liver

Gastrointestinal infection, gastritis, and liver disorders Strongly bitter and detoxifying, goldenseal exerts a positive influence on the stomach, intestines, and liver, helping in conditions as varied as peptic ulcer, dysbiosis, candidiasis, chronic gastroenteritis, and hepatitis.

Chronic infection Goldenseal can significantly boost the body's ability to resist and shrug off lingering infection, whether it is a local fungal infection or glandular fever. It is often combined with echinacea (*Echinacea purpurea*).

Native to North American woodlands, goldenseal is threatened in the wild through overharvesting. Use cultivated, organic root only.

Congestion problems Goldenseal improves the health of mucous membranes. It is useful, for example, in sinus and middle ear congestion, particularly where linked to chronic infection, as well in vaginal infection, where local application of a decoction may be helpful.

root contains alkaloids with strong antimicrobial activity

FRESH ROOT

KEY INFORMATION

SAFETY	★ ★ ★ ½ ☆
TRADITIONAL USE	★ ★ ★ ★ ★
RESEARCH	★ ★ ★ ½ ☆

BEST TAKEN AS Tincture ✓✓✓ Tablet ✓✓ Capsule ✓
DOSAGE C (*see pp.44–45*)
OFTEN USED WITH Echinacea (*Echinacea purpurea*)
CAUTIONS Do not take during pregnancy and while breast-feeding. Not suitable for children. Keep to recommended dosage—high doses can irritate mucous membranes. See also pp.42–51.

St. John's wort

Hypericum perforatum

Few herbs are as well-known as St. John's wort, its popularity resulting from conclusive clinical research and first-hand experience of its effectiveness in treating mild to moderate depression. Other uses include seasonal affective disorder, jet lag, and nervous exhaustion.

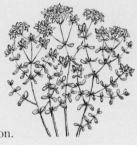

MEDICINAL USES

Part used   Flowering top

Key actions   Antidepressant ● Antiviral ● Nerve tonic ● Wound healer

Depression, disturbed sleep, seasonal affective disorder (SAD) Constituents of St. John's wort influence brain chemistry in several different ways, leading to better mood and morale. Sleep, vitality, and the ability to relax may also improve. Positive results may take up to six weeks; more commonly, improvement starts within two weeks. The herb helps banish the "winter blues," reducing the impact of SAD during the winter months. In European herbal medicine, St. John's wort has always been seen as a remedy to drive away down-heartedness and to heal wounds, and these areas remain its core therapeutic uses. Clinical trials indicate that side effects from taking St. John's wort are mild and very infrequent. Risks in taking it arise only when it is used

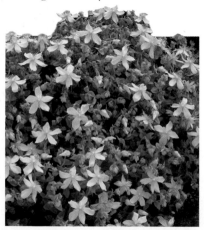

KEY INFORMATION

SAFETY	★ ★ ★ ★ ☆
TRADITIONAL USE	★ ★ ★ ★ ☆
RESEARCH	★ ★ ★ ★ ★

BEST. TAKEN AS Tincture ✓✓✓ Infusion ✓✓ Tablet, capsule, fixed oil (topically) ✓

DOSAGE M, C (*see pp.44–45*)

OFTEN USED WITH Valerian (*Valeriana officinalis*)

CAUTIONS Can cause sensitivity to sunlight. If taking prescribed medication, including oral contraceptives, seek advice from an herbal or medical practitioner before commencing treatment with St. John's wort. Do not combine with other antidepressants. See also pp.42–51.

flowering tops are used to lift mood and morale

DRIED FLOWERS

alongside certain conventional medicines since, by stimulating liver detoxification, St. John's wort lowers drug levels within the body and thus reduces their effectiveness. In practice, this means that if taking prescribed medication, you should seek advice from an herbal practitioner or doctor before taking St. John's wort.

Anxiety, nervous exhaustion Although emphasis is placed on the herb's ability to relieve depression, it also works well in relaxing and strengthening an exhausted nervous system that can occur as a result of long-term stress or worry. It can be particularly beneficial in cases involving

St. John's wort takes its name from the fact that the herb traditionally flowers by, and is harvested around, St. John's Day on June 24th.

ST. JOHN'S WORT OIL

To make the oil, collect the flowering tops of St. John's wort on a dry, sunny morning. Carefully chop the herb material into ⅓in (1cm) lengths and place in a large clear glass jar. Pour organic olive oil overtop until the herb is fully covered. Stir the contents thoroughly and seal. Put on a sunny windowsill and leave for four weeks until the oil turns pale crimson. Strain and bottle, or for a stronger oil repeat, using a fresh batch of herb.

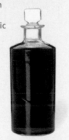

FIXED OIL

both anxiety and depression. St. John's wort can help lift mood and vitality during menopause, while its effect on the hormone melatonin may make it useful for jetlag.

St. John's wort has dark red oil glands that line the margins of both petals and leaves. These glands contain hypericin, a key active constituent.

Toothache, sciatica, shingles St. John's wort oil helps to dull nerve pain and speed tissue repair. Apply fixed oil directly on the skin overlying neuralgic areas or apply on the cheek before dental treatment.

Gastritis and stomach ulcer, local wound healing The herb's wound-healing properties can be put to good use, whether taken internally or applied externally. For stomach ulcers, take one teaspoonful of fixed oil a day. The fixed oil, which is naturally antiseptic, is traditionally regarded as useful for knife and puncture wounds, and aids healing of wounds, sprains, bruises, and arthritic joints. The oil can also be applied to post-operative scars—a modern extension of its traditional use. Essential oils may be added to the oil for topical use, as required.

dark red oil glands

Elecampane

Inula helenium

Before the development of modern antibiotics, elecampane was one of the principal medicines available for treating tuberculosis. Rarely effective in treating such deep-seated infection, elecampane is nevertheless an effective and well-tolerated remedy for coughs and chest conditions such as bronchitis.

MEDICINAL USES

Part used Root

Key actions Antibacterial ● Diaphoretic (induces sweating) ● Expectorant ● Mild bitter ● Tonic

Cough, chest infection, and congestion
Elecampane helps relieve both dry irritable and wet congested coughs. Best combined with other cough remedies, for example thyme (*Thymus vulgaris*), it may be safely given to children with chest coughs. Its antibacterial action helps disinfect the lungs, while congested phlegm is shifted and more readily coughed up. Elecampane combines well with remedies such as elderflower (*Sambucus nigra*) for congestion in the ear, nose, and throat, particularly where catarrh is dripping down the throat into the bronchial tubes. It can also prove useful in bronchial asthma.

Convalescence With a tonic action on both respiratory and digestive systems, elecampane makes a first-rate remedy for convalescence, improving appetite and restoring vitality, especially after a chest infection. The warm decoction, taken routinely throughout the winter, will help to protect against recurrence of infection.

Gastrointestinal parasites Elecampane has notable activity against intestinal worms and parasites. In combination with other remedies, it has been used successfully to treat amebic dysentery.

A vigorous perennial growing up to 10ft (3m) in height, elecampane has deep roots that are harvested and dried in autumn.

KEY INFORMATION

SAFETY	★ ★ ★ ★ ⯪
TRADITIONAL USE	★ ★ ★ ★ ☆
RESEARCH	★ ★ ★⯪ ☆

BEST TAKEN AS Tincture ✓✓✓ Decoction ✓✓ Tablet, Capsule ✓
DOSAGE B (*see pp.44–45*)
OFTEN USED WITH Licorice (*Glycyrrhiza glabra*)
CAUTIONS Rarely, can cause allergic reaction or gastrointestinal upset. Not advised in pregnancy and while breast-feeding. See also pp.42–51.

FRESH ROOT

Shiitake

Lentinus edodes

Reputedly given to the Japanese emperor in 199CE, shiitake mushroom has been used in traditional medicine for centuries as a tonic and restorative remedy, often for severe and chronic illness. Recent research suggests that shiitake extract has promise as an anticancer remedy.

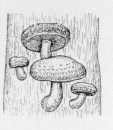

MEDICINAL USES

Part used Fungi

Key actions Antitumor ● Antiviral ● Immune-enhancing ● Protects liver

Anticancer remedy Following extensive Japanese research, fairly high doses of shiitake extract are recommended in cancer treatment, lower dose long-term treatment being used to support immune function and act as a cancer preventative. As an anticancer agent, shiitake appears to be most effective when taken alongside chemotherapy, the extract acting to stimulate programmed cell death and to protect the liver and immune system from toxic damage. In this situation, shiitake extract should only be taken on the advice of a suitably experienced herbal practitioner or doctor.

Other uses Many chronic health problems such as viral hepatitis, chronic fatigue syndrome, candidiasis, and recurrent infections can benefit from shiitake's positive

makes "medicinal" soup

DRIED MUSHROOMS

action on immune function. Shiitake can also be taken to maintain good health, especially in old age. For medicinal use, take shiitake extract. Shiitake mushrooms make a good addition to a healthy diet.

Shiitake grows naturally on fallen broadleaf trees in temperate regions of eastern Asia, including China and Japan. It is now widely cultivated in the West.

KEY INFORMATION

SAFETY   ★ ★ ★ ★ ☆
TRADITIONAL USE   ★ ★ ★ ★ ★
RESEARCH   ★ ★ ★ ⯪ ☆
BEST TAKEN AS Standardized extract, fungi (as food) ✓✓✓
DOSAGE M, Food (*see pp.44–45*)
OFTEN USED WITH Reishi mushroom (*Ganoderma lucida*)
CAUTIONS Can cause diarrhea and allergic skin reactions, as well as elevation of blood counts. See also pp.42–51.

Lavender

Lavandula angustifolia, L. officinalis, L. vera

Lavender combines beauty and function, delicate aroma with great therapeutic use, and an exceptional safety record. Its dried flowers and essential oil revive the spirits and at the same time earn a place in every home's first aid kit. Little wonder that lavender is so popular.

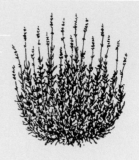

MEDICINAL USES

Parts used Essential oil ● Flower ● Leaves

Key actions Analgesic ● Antidepressant ● Antiseptic● Antispasmodic ● Relieves gas ● Sedative

Anxiety, irritability, headache Anxiety and tension are key words for lavender, its calming qualities soothing nervous overactivity, stress-related headache, and migraine. Lavender combines well with rosemary (*Rosmarinus officinalis*) to alleviate nervous exhaustion and improve weak circulation. It is also known to have mood-enhancing properties. This combination of mild sedative and antidepressant activity makes it particularly suitable where lowered mood and vitality follow long-term worry or overactivity.

Sleep difficulties Used as essential oil (a few drops placed on an oil burner or used in a massage), dried flowers (in an herb pillow), or as a tincture (a teaspoon before going to bed), lavender improves sleep quality and the

KEY INFORMATION

SAFETY	★ ★ ★ ★ ★
TRADITIONAL USE	★ ★ ★ ★ ★
RESEARCH	★ ★ ★ ⯪ ☆

BEST TAKEN AS Essential oil (topically) ✓✓✓ Tincture ✓✓ Infusion ✓
DOSAGE B (*see pp.44–45*)
OFTEN USED WITH Rosemary (*Rosmarinus officinalis*)
CAUTIONS Rarely, when applied topically, the oil can cause contact dermatitis. Do not take the essential oil internally. See also pp.42–51.

chance of a good night's sleep. It combines well with other herbal sleep remedies, notably passion flower (*Passiflora incarnata*) and lemon balm (*Melissa officinalis*).

Local pain relief and relaxation Lavender oil can be applied to the skin in almost any situation involving pain. Massage the oil onto herpes or shingles sores, rheumatic joints, the cheek overlying an aching tooth, or the forehead and temples for a migraine. A few drops of oil on a cotton ball plugged into the ear relieves a mild earache. Lavender tincture or tea can provide systemic support, helping relax tensed and aching muscles. For menstrual cramps and pain, tincture or tea taken internally and oil massaged into the lower abdomen can bring quick relief.

Digestive problems Most often combined with other digestive remedies, lavender has specific value where emotional distress is the underlying cause of digestive disturbance such as "butterflies" in the stomach, bloating, belching, and irritable bowel symptoms.

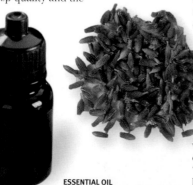

ESSENTIAL OIL

Other uses In France, lavender is used in the treatment of a wide range of respiratory problems, including flu, cough, whooping cough, asthma, and bronchitis. Its antispasmodic and antiseptic activity combines well with other herbs such as thyme (*Thymus vulgaris*) and elecampane (*Inula helenium*). The flowers are sometimes used as a gargle for painful and inflamed sore throat; in this situation, lavender combines well with licorice (*Glycyrrhiza glabra*). Lavender tea or tincture has long-standing use as a tonic for weak and nervy children; since neither taste as good as they smell, they can be diluted in unsweetened blackcurrant or apple juice.

aromatic flower heads are antispasmodic and mildly sedative

Native to France and the western Mediterranean, lavender is cultivated worldwide for its volatile oil.

LAVENDER—THE ESSENTIAL OIL

Possibly the only essential oil that is safe to apply neat to large areas of the skin, lavender oil is a key first aid remedy for home use and when traveling. A few drops massaged into the temples or the back of the neck can bring swift relief to headache and neck and shoulder tension. Aches and pains elsewhere in the body will also benefit. Apply the oil to minor burns, sunburn, sores, itchy skin problems, and insect bites and stings, to promote healing and ease discomfort. The oil also makes a reasonably effective insect repellent.

PAIN RELIEF

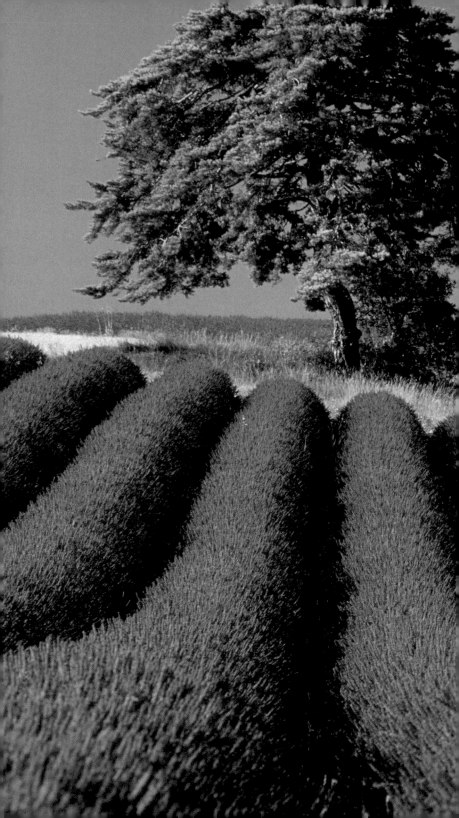

Aromatic and relaxing, lavender (*Lavandula officinalis*) is cultivated widely for its medicinal properties. Its healing and pain-relieving essential oil is a favorite first aid remedy.

Motherwort

Leonorus cardiaca

An undervalued remedy, motherwort has an unusual combination of actions, all tending to calm those with a nervous disposition, while strengthening cardiovascular and digestive function. The herb's botanical name indicates its longstanding use as a remedy for an irregular or fast heartbeat.

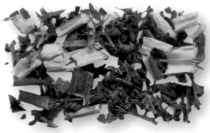

MEDICINAL USES

Part used Flowering top

Key actions Aids menstruation ● Heart tonic ● Lowers blood pressure ● Mild bitter ● Nerve tonic ● Relaxant

Menstrual problems Used to promote a regular and symptom-free menstrual cycle, motherwort relieves premenstrual tension and period pains. It stimulates the onset of menstruation, and is also

DRIED AERIAL PARTS

helpful where an irregular or absent menstrual cycle is linked to poor appetite or low body weight.

Heart and thyroid problems
Motherwort is a key remedy for palpitations and irregular heartbeat, especially when they are linked with anxiety or an overactive thyroid. Small, frequent doses (a few drops of tincture) can sometimes be sufficient to control such problems. It is prescribed by herbal practitioners for angina, coronary heart disease, and high blood pressure.

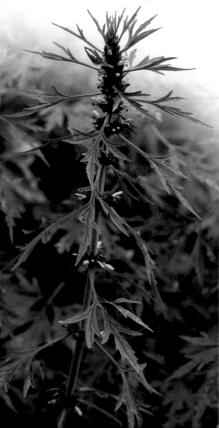

Used for centuries to treat heart palpitations, motherwort, a perennial herb, grows in much of Europe and North America.

KEY INFORMATION

SAFETY	★ ★ ★ ★ ☆
TRADITIONAL USE	★ ★ ★ ★ ☆
RESEARCH	★ ★ ☆ ☆ ☆

BEST TAKEN AS Infusion ✓✓✓
Tincture ✓✓ Capsule ✓
DOSAGE C (*see pp.44–45*)
OFTEN USED WITH Cramp bark (*Viburnum opulus*)
CAUTIONS Do not take during pregnancy. Avoid in heavy menstrual bleeding. See also pp.42–51.

Lemon verbena

Lippia citriodora syn. *Aloysia triphylla*

Native to South America, lemon verbena is best used as a refreshing tea. It has sedative and relaxant properties, and can be used as an insect repellent.

MEDICINAL USES

Part used Leaf ● Flowers

Key actions Antispasmodic ● Sedative

Sleep difficulties The gentle-acting infusion of lemon verbena leaves makes a pleasant after-dinner and late-evening drink, aiding relaxation and helping to prevent insomnia and restlessness. The herb has a mild tonic effect on the nervous system, which lifts the spirits and helps counter depression.

Digestive aid The lemon-scented volatile oil in the infusion improves digestion and soothes discomfort in the stomach, calming gas and bloating.

KEY INFORMATION

SAFETY	★ ★ ★ ★ ☆
TRADITIONAL USE	★ ★ ★ ☆ ☆
RESEARCH	★ ★ ☆ ☆ ☆
BEST TAKEN AS	Infusion ✓✓✓
DOSAGE	C (*see pp.44–45*)
CAUTIONS	None known. See also pp.42–51.

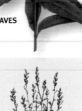

FRESH LEAVES

Lobelia

Lobelia inflata

A valuable remedy in the treatment of respiratory problems, lobelia is potentially toxic and should be taken only when prescribed or as a licensed medicine.

MEDICINAL USES

Parts used Aerial parts

KEY INFORMATION

SAFETY	★ ★ ☆ ☆ ☆
TRADITIONAL USE	★ ★ ★ ★ ★
RESEARCH	★ ★ ☆ ☆ ☆
BEST TAKEN AS	Over-the-counter remedy ✓✓✓
DOSAGE	M (*see pp.44–45*)
CAUTIONS	May cause vomiting in high dosage. Take only when prescribed by an herbal or medical practitioner, or when part of a licensed over-the-counter medicine. Restricted herb in some countries, including Australia. See also pp.42–51.

Key actions Antispasmodic ● Expectorant ● Stimulates breathing

Chest complaints Lobelia relaxes the airways, stimulates coughing up of mucus, and eases wheezing in the chest. It promotes deeper and stronger breathing and is a valuable remedy for tight-chested conditions such as asthma and chronic bronchitis.

FLOWERS AND LEAVES

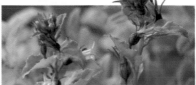

Linseed, Flax

Linum usitatissimum

Grown as a food crop in temperate climates, linseed, or flax, is a valuable and readily available dietary supplement. A rich source of protein and omega-3 oils, linseed also contains high levels of phytoestrogens—roughly 10 times more than other seeds, making it a key remedy for menopause.

MEDICINAL USES

Part used Seed

Key actions Antioxidant • Demulcent • Estrogenic • Laxative • Nutritive

Food supplement, menopausal symptoms Ground or cracked seed (untreated seed is not absorbed) makes an excellent addition to the diet: take 1–2 tablespoons a day with muesli, breakfast cereal, or yogurt. Since the seed soaks up large quantities of liquid, drink a large glass of water at the same time. The a-linoleic acid and omega-3 oil content in the seed is similar to fish oils, although less biologically available. High levels of phytoestrogens make linseed a useful supplement for menopausal symptoms such as hot flashes and headache. Store ground or cracked seed in an airtight container in the refrigerator to prevent the seed oils going rancid. Use within two to three weeks.

Digestive problems An excellent bulk laxative, linseed is a safe and frequently effective remedy for chronic constipation. Soak 1 tablespoonful of seed in at least

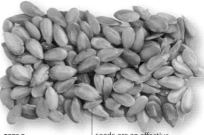

SEEDS | seeds are an effective remedy for constipation

5 times its volume of warm water. Leave for a few hours, then swallow, preferably drinking additional water. The resulting jelly-like brew will often prove helpful for constipation and can also relieve acid indigestion and diarrhea. Long-term problems such as acid reflux and esophagitis, peptic ulcer, and chronic constipation are likely to need ongoing treatment with linseed.

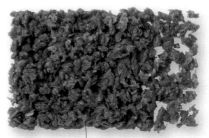

CRUSHED SEEDS | crushed seeds are a rich source of omega-3 fatty acids

Respiratory disorders Taken in the form of soaked seed as described for digestive problems (*see above*), linseed soothes the chest and airways and can prove helpful in conditions such as chronic or irritable coughs, hoarseness, bronchitis, pleurisy, and emphysema.

KEY INFORMATION

SAFETY	★ ★ ★ ★ ☆
TRADITIONAL USE	★ ★ ★ ★ ☆
RESEARCH	★ ★ ★ ★ ☆

BEST TAKEN AS Ground or cracked seed ✓✓✓

DOSAGE 1–2 tablespoons a day, with plenty of water.

CAUTIONS Always dilute with at least 5 times the volume of water. Unripe seed can be toxic. See also pp.42–51.

The seed may also be applied to the chest wall as a poultice (*see Topical use, below*) to relieve congestive bronchitis.

Topical use Linseed also finds use when applied locally to the skin as a poultice. Put warm soaked seed in gauze or muslin and hold or bind in place on burns, bites and stings, boils, and hemorrhoids. A warm poultice can also be used to "draw" splinters and boils, the mucilage in the seed soaking up fluids and waste products.

Other uses Although research is so far not conclusive, there are indications that linseed can prove to be a useful remedy in a remarkably wide range of serious health problems. It appears to have a soothing effect on the kidneys and may be helpful in kidney disease. Within the gut it helps to prevent absorption of fats and sugars, and makes a good addition in both cholesterol-lowering regimes and diet-controlled diabetes. Partly as a result of its high phytoestrogen content, linseed appears to have important cancer-preventative activity, particularly against estrogen-dependent cancers such as breast cancer. It is thought to reduce re-absorption of estrogens within the colon, and is likely to prove useful in the treatment of colon cancer. In the above conditions, use linseed only after consulting your doctor or herbal practitioner.

LINSEED OR FLAX OIL

Flax or linseed oil contains uniquely high levels (typically around 55 percent) of a-linolenic acid, an omega-3 polyunsaturated fatty acid similar to those found in fish oils. Plant-derived omega-3 oils are not so readily available for use by the body as fish oils, but nevertheless provide similar health benefits. All omega-3 oils have a protective activity on the heart and circulation and against cancer.

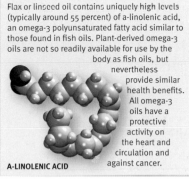

A-LINOLENIC ACID

Cultivated for food in Africa since 5000–8000 BCE, linseed was first brought to North America for its stem fiber to make linen and paper.

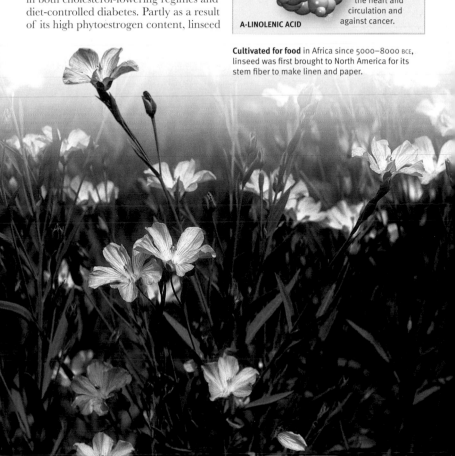

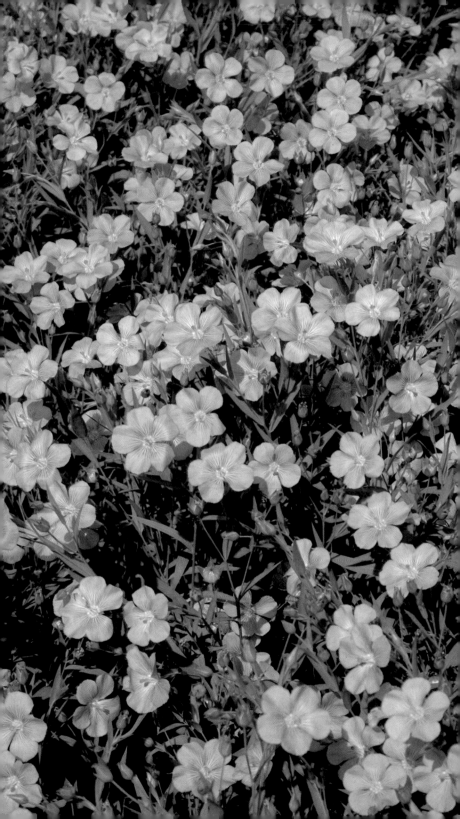

With longstanding medicinal as well as industrial use, linseed (*Linum usitatissimum*) is better known today as the main vegetable source of omega-3 essential fatty acids.

Alfalfa, Lucerne

Medicago sativa

Most used as animal feed, alfalfa is equally nutritious for humans, containing appreciable levels of protein, calcium, magnesium, vitamins C, E, K, and beta-carotene. Its main traditional use has been as a natural food supplement for debility and convalescence, aiding appetite and weight gain.

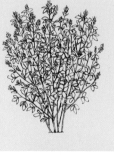

MEDICINAL USES

Parts used Aerial parts ● Sprout

Key actions Appetite stimulant ● Estrogenic ● Nutritive ● Stimulates breast milk

Convalescence and debility Alfalfa infusion and sprouts provide high-quality and easily absorbed nutrition, especially when taken medium-term. Indications for their use include poor appetite, convalescence, inability to gain weight, and anorexia nervosa.

Menopausal symptoms Alfalfa is a useful food to supplement during menopause. Unlike soya, it does not inhibit the absorption of minerals such as iron and calcium. Alfalfa contains

With easily assimilated nutrients, alfalfa's combination of phytoestrogens, calcium, and magnesium can prove useful in the prevention of osteoporosis.

seeds contain estrogenic isoflavones

SEEDS

estrogenic isoflavones, which have led to its recent use for menopausal symptoms, especially in combination with sage (*Salvia officinalis*).

Other uses This plant is also useful for arthritic and rheumatic symptoms, diabetes, and raised cholesterol levels.

KEY INFORMATION

SAFETY	★ ★ ★ ★ ☆
TRADITIONAL USE	★ ★ ★ ⯪ ☆
RESEARCH	★ ★ ★ ☆ ☆

BEST TAKEN AS Sprout ✓✓
Leaf infusion ✓✓✓
DOSAGE M, A, food (*see pp.44–45*)
OFTEN USED WITH Sage (*Salvia officinalis*)
CAUTIONS Keep to recommended dosage. Do not eat excessive amounts of sprouting seeds. Avoid during pregnancy. See also pp.42–51.

Tea tree

Melaleuca alternifolia

In aboriginal medicine, tea tree leaves, crushed and inhaled or infused, were employed to treat infections of all kinds. Today, the essential oil is normally used, its unrivaled antiseptic action proving effective at countering fungal infection affecting the hair, skin, and nails.

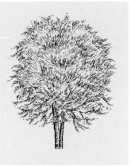

MEDICINAL USES

Parts used Essential oil • Leaf

Key actions Antifungal • Antiseptic

Skin infections A must-have for any home herbal first aid kit, tea tree oil can help treat many minor fungal and bacterial skin problems. On boils, acne spots, and small patches of fungal infection, like an affected toenail, apply neat tea tree oil sparingly twice a day. For larger areas, apply tea tree oil diluted in calendula (*Calendula officinalis*) or wheatgerm (*Triticum vulgare*) oil. Combine 1 part tea tree oil to 10 parts carrier oil and massage onto the affected area.

Ear infection For infection of the external ear passage and for a mild earache, put 1–2 drops of neat oil on cotton wool and plug into the affected ear overnight. Tea tree oil combines well with lavender oil   use 1 drop of each.

Vaginal infection For vaginal infections such as thrush, diluted tea tree oil can be applied to the affected area, although it is likely to sting. It is far better to use tea tree suppositories. Insert one every night for 3–4 days, stop for a few days, and then start again as required.

KEY INFORMATION

SAFETY	★★★★☆
TRADITIONAL USE	★★★★★
RESEARCH	★★★★☆

BEST TAKEN AS Neat or diluted essential oil (topical) ✓✓✓ Suppository ✓✓
DOSAGE T (*see pp.44–45*)
OFTEN USED WITH Calendula fixed oil
CAUTIONS Do not take essential oil internally. Can occasionally cause dermatitis with topical preparations. See also pp.42–51.

Native to Australia, tea tree flourishes in moist soils in northern New South Wales and Queensland. The leaves are distilled to produce the essential oil.

leaves are a natural insect repellent

leaves contain highly antiseptic volatile oil

FRESH LEAVES

Lemon balm, Melissa

Melissa officinalis

Much loved as a lemon-scented infusion that "makes the heart merry", lemon balm's soothing qualities quiet the heart and an overactive mind. Valuable in situations where long-term anxiety edges into depression, lemon balm is known to inhibit thyroid function and makes a useful remedy for a slightly overactive thyroid gland.

MEDICINAL USES

Part used Leaf

Key actions Antidepressant
- Antispasmodic ● Insect repellent
- Relaxant ● Relieves gas
- Topical (antiviral)

Anxiety, tension headache, insomnia, palpitations Lemon balm is a relaxing tonic for anxiety, mild depression, restlessness, and insomnia. It reduces feelings of panic and is a valuable remedy for palpitations of a nervous origin. For all such conditions, take as an infusion or tincture 2–3 times a day with

leaves are used as an insect repellent

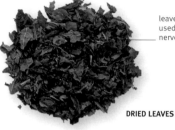

leaves are used as a nerve tonic

DRIED LEAVES

additional doses if required. Lemon balm combines well with skullcap (*Scutellaria lateriflora*).

Colic, gas, bloating Safe for children, lemon balm infusion helps to relieve spasmodic pains and is specifically used for stress-related stomach disorders such as acidity, indigestion, colicky pain, gas, and bloating.

Other uses An infusion or tincture can be applied to speed the healing of cold sores or dabbed on as an insect repellent. The herb will help in mild hyperthyroid states, especially when the heartbeat is irregular or too fast.

With an aromatic and pleasant bitter-lemon taste, lemon balm is a common ingredient in liqueurs and *digestifs*, including Benedictine.

KEY INFORMATION

SAFETY	★ ★ ★ ★ ★
TRADITIONAL USE	★ ★ ★ ★ ☆
RESEARCH	★ ★ ★ ☆ ☆

BEST TAKEN AS Infusion
(fresh leaves) ✓✓✓ Tincture ✓✓
DOSAGE C (*see pp.44–45*)
OFTEN USED WITH Rosemary
(*Rosmarinus officinalis*)
CAUTIONS None known. See also pp.42–51.

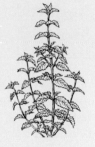

Peppermint

Mentha x piperita

A mint hybrid first grown in England in the 17th century, peppermint is known around the world for its cool and flavorful taste. Commonly taken after a meal to aid digestion, the infusion is a useful remedy for flatulence and bloating as well as headaches and migraines linked to digestive weakness.

MEDICINAL USES

Parts used Leaf ● Essential oil

Key actions Antiseptic ● Antispasmodic ● Diaphoretic ● Relieves gas ● Mild analgesic ● Mild sedative ● Mild bitter

Gas, nausea, cramps, irritable bowel

Clinical research confirms the usefulness of peppermint essential oil in irritable bowel syndrome. The essential oil acts on the colon, relieving spasm and irritability, and reducing the sensitivity of nerve endings in the intestinal wall. The milder-acting infusion can be safely taken for symptoms such as bad breath, gas, belching, bloating, and colic.

Colds, flu, headache, migraine

Peppermint and elderflower (*Sambucus nigra*) make an effective combination for fever, colds, catarrh, and gastric infection. Hot peppermint tea encourages sweating and cools fever. Drink tea or apply 1–2 drops of peppermint oil to forehead to relieve headache and migraine.

Topical uses Peppermint oil is soothing for itchy skin. Apply at 2 percent dilution (2 drops per teaspoonful of carrier oil) to affected areas. The infusion can be applied as a lotion to relieve nettle rash and eczema. Be careful to avoid the eyes.

KEY INFORMATION

SAFETY	★★★★☆
TRADITIONAL USE	★★★★⯪
RESEARCH	★★★★☆

BEST TAKEN AS Infusion ✓✓✓
Tincture ✓✓ Enteric-coated capsules (with prescription only) ✓
DOSAGE C (*see pages 44–45*)
OFTEN USED WITH Elderflower (*Sambucus nigra*).
CAUTIONS Do not give to children under the age of 5. Essential oil is best taken internally on the recommendation of an herbal or medical practitioner. See also pp.42–51.

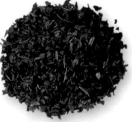

INFUSION

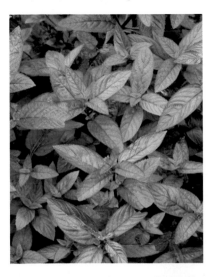

Peppermint leaf makes a good after-dinner drink.

DRIED AERIAL PARTS

Bogbean

Menyanthes trifoliata

Strongly bitter, bogbean is mostly used to improve a weak or underactive digestive system or to treat rheumatic symptoms, whether resulting from local or systemic inflammation. It is a threatened species because its natural habitat is disappearing; use organic products.

MEDICINAL USES

Part used Leaf

Key actions Antirheumatic ● Bitter tonic ● Laxative (large doses)

Arthritic, rheumatic, and kidney problems Generally prescribed by herbal practitioners rather than self-medicated, bogbean can provide relief in conditions as varied as fibromyalgia, gout, polymyalgia rheumatica, and rheumatoid arthritis. Seen as a specific for muscular, rather than joint, aches and pains, it combines well with other antirheumatic herbs, including birch (*Betula alba*) and celery (*Apium graveolens*). It has a reputation of supporting kidney clearance of waste products and has been used in kidney disease.

Loss of appetite, weak digestion

Bogbean stimulates appetite and the flow of saliva and digestive juices, leading to better processing of foods and absorption of nutrients. An irritant laxative at high doses, it should be avoided where the bowels are loose or sensitive, such as in irritable bowel syndrome.

leaves have a strong bitter taste

DRIED LEAVES

Unglamorously but accurately named, bogbean thrives in boggy, marshy places and fresh shallow water.

KEY INFORMATION

SAFETY   ★ ★ ★ ★ ☆
TRADITIONAL USE   ★ ★ ★ ⯨ ☆
RESEARCH   ★ ★ ⯨ ☆ ☆
BEST TAKEN AS Tincture ✓ ✓ ✓
DOSAGE C (*see pp.44–45*)
OFTEN USED WITH Celery seed (*Apium graveolens*)
CAUTIONS May cause diarrhea. Avoid during pregnancy and while breast-feeding. See also pp.42–51.

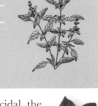

Basil

Ocimum basilicum

The herb in Italian cooking, basil relieves upper digestive discomfort, indigestion, and bloating, and is applied topically to acne and insect bites.

MEDICINAL USES

Part used Whole plant

Key actions Antibacterial ● Insecticidal ● Mild sedative ● Relieves gas

Digestive problems Like many culinary herbs, basil has a pronounced effect on digestion, both stimulating and soothing stomach and intestinal activity at the same time. It is best taken for symptoms such as bad breath, stomach cramps, nausea, indigestion, gas, and bloating.

Other uses Juice from the leaves can be applied neat to infected spots and insect bites and stings to speed healing.

Significantly insecticidal, the leaves or juice can be rubbed on the skin to repel insects.

AERIAL PARTS

KEY INFORMATION

SAFETY	★★★★☆
TRADITIONAL USE	★★★⯪☆
RESEARCH	★★★☆☆

BEST TAKEN AS Infusion ✓✓✓ Capsule ✓✓ Food ✓
DOSAGE C *(see pp.44–45)*
CAUTIONS Safe at recommended dosage. See also pp.42–51.

Holy basil, Tulsi

Ocimum sanctum

Prized in Indian medicine as a tonic that clears the mind, holy basil has many benefits, including stabilizing blood sugar levels and soothing chest conditions.

MEDICINAL USES

Part used Whole plant

Key actions Anti-inflammatory ● Expectorant ● Lowers blood sugar levels ● Tonic

FRESH LEAVES

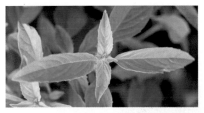

Uses Holy basil promotes better uptake of sugars within the body, and can prove particularly helpful in the early stages of diabetes. Commonly used for cough and bronchitis, holy basil also helps to lower blood pressure and cholesterol.

KEY INFORMATION

SAFETY	★★★★☆
TRADITIONAL USE	★★★★★
RESEARCH	★★★★☆

BEST TAKEN AS Infusion ✓✓✓ Tincture ✓✓ Powder ✓
DOSAGE C *(see pp.44–45)*
CAUTIONS In diabetes, take only after consulting a professional. See also pp.42–51.

A prolific flowering herb, evening primrose (*Oenothera biennis*) produces thousands of seeds, several hundred of which need to be pressed for just one capsule of seed oil.

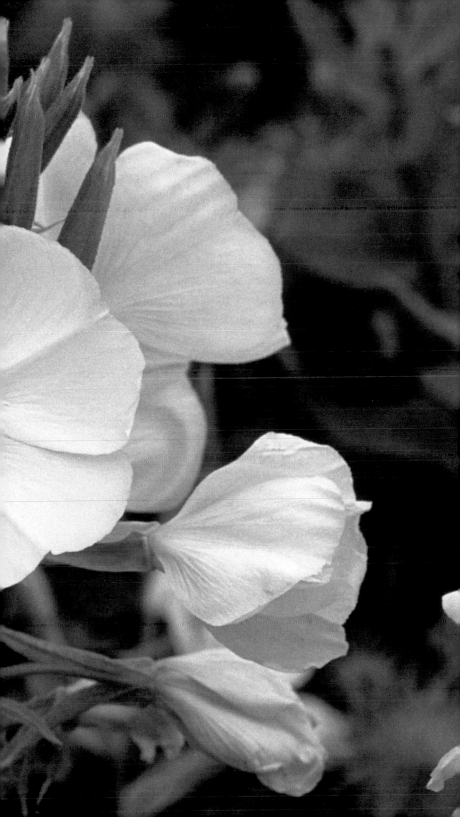

Evening primrose

Oenothera biennis

Researched in England since the 1980s, evening primrose seed oil (EPO) is high in omega-6 essential fatty acids and can prove helpful in a range of inflammatory conditions, such as menstrual problems, rheumatoid arthritis, and eczema. It is thought to work in two distinct ways to block inflammatory processes.

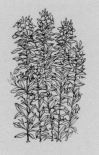

MEDICINAL USES

Parts used Seed • Seed oil

Key actions Anti-inflammatory • Antioxidant • Emollient

Skin conditions Less concentrated than borage oil but with similar therapeutic effects, EPO makes a useful supplement for eczema and dermatitis. It is considered safe for infants as well. For best results, take internally for several months and apply topically to affected areas of skin.

Menstrual disorders Studies show that EPO can bring relief to premenstrual syndrome (PMS), especially where breast or menstrual pain are key problems. In both cases, EPO is best combined with a vitamin B complex supplement.

KEY INFORMATION

SAFETY	★ ★ ★ ★ ★
TRADITIONAL USE	★ ★ ★ ☆ ☆
RESEARCH	★ ★ ★ ★ ☆

BEST TAKEN AS Capsule ✓✓✓
Oil (topically) ✓✓
DOSAGE M (*see pp.44–45*)
OFTEN USED WITH Vitamin E
CAUTIONS Safe at recommended dosage. Avoid during pregnancy. Take only after consulting an herbal or medical practitioner if taking epilepsy medication. See also pp.42–51.

SEED-OIL CAPSULE

Inflammation EPO can act to reduce inflammation in chronic inflammatory disease, easing symptoms in joints and muscles, such as in rheumatoid arthritis. EPO can also help ease the discomfort of dry eyes and deficient skin secretion in Sjögren's syndrome.

Grown commercially for its seed oil, evening primrose is a native of North America and thrives on wasteland, especially in sandy soil.

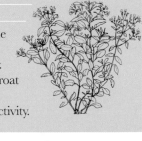

Oregano, Wild marjoram

Origanum majorana, O. vulgare

Common to cuisines of the Mediterranean, the aromatic, slightly spicy flavor of oregano adds zest to food, while stimulating digestive activity. The herb is used for digestive disorders and throat or chest infections. Essential oils from oregano species have strong antiseptic and antifungal activity.

MEDICINAL USES

Parts used Aerial parts ● Essential oil

Key actions Antifungal ● Antioxidant ● Antiseptic ● Expectorant ● Stimulant

Respiratory and digestive infection

With strongly antiseptic and anti-microbial constituents, oregano infusion or tincture is a useful expectorant in bronchial infection, chesty coughs, and respiratory catarrh. Digestive problems such as gastroenteritis and candida infection will also benefit from the herb's tonic activity, especially where bloating and food intolerance are present. For mouth and throat infections, including oral thrush, use the infusion as a mouthwash or gargle, then swallow.

Other uses Apply the infusion or the diluted oil (a maximum of 5 percent dilution in a carrier oil such as olive oil) regularly to skin problems such as ringworm and fungal nails.

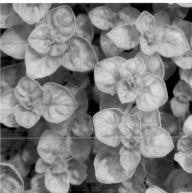

An upright perennial with aromatic, oval leaves, oregano or cultivated marjoram is a common kitchen garden herb, used often in Mediterranean cooking.

wild plant is weaker in action than garden varieties

DRIED LEAVES AND FLOWERS

KEY INFORMATION

SAFETY	★ ★ ★ ★ ☆
TRADITIONAL USE	★ ★ ★ ★ ☆
RESEARCH	★ ☆ ☆ ☆ ☆

BEST TAKEN AS Infusion ✓✓✓ Tincture ✓✓ Capsule ✓

DOSAGE C (*see pp.44–45*)

OFTEN USED WITH Olive leaf (*Olea europeae*)

CAUTIONS Do not take during pregnancy. Do not take essential oil internally unless recommended by a herbal or medical practitioner. Can cause skin irritation and gastrointestinal upset. See also pp.42–51.

WILD MARJORAM

White peony

Paeonia lactiflora

A traditional Chinese remedy taken to cool excess heat, white peony is mostly used in the West for period pains, menstrual irregularity, and fibroids.

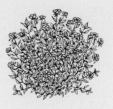

MEDICINAL USES

Part used Root

Key actions Anti-inflammatory ● Antispasmodic ● Tonic

Gynecological problems Although it is taken most often to ease period pains and to treat fibroids, when combined with licorice (*Glycyrrhiza glabra*), white peony acts to reverse the symptoms of polycystic ovary syndrome and may help to improve fertility in this condition.

FLOWER

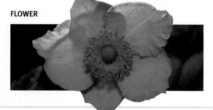

KEY INFORMATION

SAFETY   ★★★★☆
TRADITIONAL USE ★★★★☆
RESEARCH   ★★★☆☆
BEST TAKEN AS Decoction ✓✓✓ Tincture ✓✓
DOSAGE B (*see pp.44–45*)
CAUTIONS Do not take if taking prescribed blood thinners. Avoid during pregnancy. Rarely can cause gastrointestinal upset. See also pp.42–51.

Guarana

Paullinia cupana

Up to 67 percent caffeine by weight, guarana is a popular Brazilian drink used to boost alertness and energy and, by athletes, to enhance peak performance.

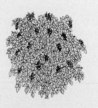

MEDICINAL USES

Part used Seed (roasted)

Key actions Antioxidant ● Astringent ● Stimulant

Low vitality and stamina Guarana is taken much like coffee to ward off fatigue, maintain attention and alertness, and to support maximum energy output, to aid in sports competition, for example. Like other caffeinated products, it can prove helpful in relieving tension headaches and migraines. It has been used symptomatically to treat diarrhea. However, it is often too stimulant for those with chronic health problems.

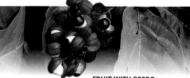

FRUIT WITH SEEDS

KEY INFORMATION

SAFETY   ★★★★☆
TRADITIONAL USE ★★★★☆
RESEARCH   ★★★☆☆
BEST TAKEN AS Tablet ✓✓✓ Drink ✓✓
DOSAGE M (*see pp.44–45*)
CAUTIONS Avoid excessive doses. Avoid if pregnant or breast-feeding. See also pp.42–51.

Passiflora, Passion flower

Passiflora incarnata

Used long before the arrival of Europeans in the Americas, passiflora's calming, relaxant qualities are quickly apparent upon taking the herb, and underlie its many uses. Passiflora is most often employed to relieve anxiety and nervousness and to aid sleep, its use in this respect confirmed by clinical trials.

MEDICINAL USES

Part used Aerial parts

Key actions Aids sleep ● Relaxant ● Relieves pain ● Sedative

Anxiety, nervousness, racing heart, headache Rarely producing drowsiness, passiflora takes the edge off worry and anxiety, bringing relief to symptoms such as a racing heart and tension headache. A mild analgesic, passiflora can help with migraines and neuralgic pain associated with toothaches, for example.

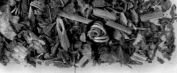

DRIED AERIAL PARTS | aerial parts are used to make relaxing infusions

Native to southern US, Central and South America, passiflora is today cultivated extensively in Europe.

Sleep disturbance, spasmodic pain Safe and non-addictive, passiflora is a key sleep remedy, often enabling one to relax and slip off into sound sleep. Its relaxant and antispasmodic activity, which is commonly overlooked, can also be used for conditions such as leg cramps and period pains.

tincture is analgesic and antispasmodic

TINCTURE

KEY INFORMATION

SAFETY ★ ★ ★ ★ ★
TRADITIONAL USE ★ ★ ★ ★ ☆
RESEARCH ★ ★ ★ ☆ ☆
BEST TAKEN AS Tincture ✓✓✓ Capsule, tablet ✓✓
DOSAGE C (*see pp.44–45*)
OFTEN USED WITH Valerian (*Valeriana officinalis*)
CAUTIONS Rarely, can cause allergic reactions. See also pp.42–51.

A key sedative remedy, passion flower (*Passiflora incarnata*) was first brought to Europe from Brazil by Jesuit priests. The complex structure of the flower was taken to signify Christ's passion.

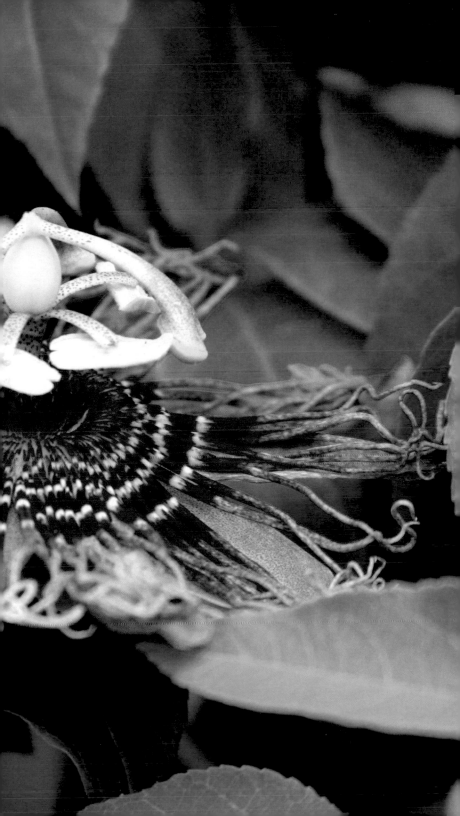

Ginseng

Panax ginseng

Ginseng has a mystique of its own, its documented use in the Far East extending back to pre-history. Taken over the centuries by kings, emperors, and popes, it has an unrivaled reputation for improving overall vitality and acting as a male tonic.

MEDICINAL USES

Part used Root

Key actions Adaptogen
● Anti-inflammatory ● Antioxidant
● Immune tonic ● Tonic

Chronic ill health, fatigue, convalescence Traditional Chinese use emphasizes ginseng's restorative qualities, helping to strengthen in depleted states and promoting longevity. Taken through the long winter months of northern China by the frail and elderly, ginseng aids physical endurance, particularly in those with lowered vitality and poor immune function. Low doses taken long-term are most likely to prove effective.

Short-term enhancement of mental and physical performance At recommended dosage, ginseng will help to increase muscle weight, physical strength, and stamina, and improve mental ability. Standard advice for healthy adults is to take for a maximum of 6 weeks. A general recommendation is to avoid caffeine while taking ginseng.

TINCTURE

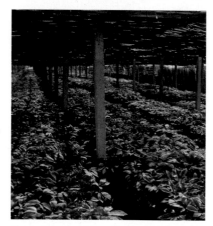

Ginseng is now rarely found in the wild. It is widely cultivated in China and Korea using intensive farming methods.

Male tonic Ginseng is probably best thought of as a male tonic rather than as an aphrodisiac. It can certainly help to improve physiological and sexual function and may also increase sexual vitality. It is the herb of choice in treating erectile dysfunction, where it combines well with ginkgo (*Ginkgo biloba*) or golden root (*Rhodiola rosea*), and for low sperm count.

Clinical trials and quality control Ginseng has been the subject of intensive research, with clinical trials investigating a wide range of potential therapeutic applications for the herb. Clinical evidence supports ginseng's use in the following ways: to enhance physical and mental performance, including coping with hunger and extremes of temperature; to improve sperm count (in

KEY INFORMATION

SAFETY	★★★★☆
TRADITIONAL USE	★★★★★
RESEARCH	★★★★☆

BEST TAKEN AS Tincture or tablet: standardized to 4% ginsenosides ✓✓✓
DOSAGE 0.5–2g a day or M (see pp.44–45)
OFTEN USED WITH Ginkgo (*Gingko biloba*)
CAUTIONS Do not take during acute illness. In high blood pressure and diabetes, consult an herbal or medical practitioner. See also pp.42–51.

THE KING OF HERBS

Regularly taken by the emperors of China and their households, ginseng's first documented use is in a Chinese herbal written 2,000 years ago: "Ginseng is a tonic to the five viscera, quieting the animal spirits, stabilizing the soul, preventing fear, expelling the vicious energies, brightening the eye, improving vision ... and prolonging life." *Shen'nong Bencaojing (Shen Nong's Materia Medica)*, 1st century CE.

CHINESE EMPEROR

Other uses Ginseng is most likely to prove helpful in treating chronic infection and a depleted immune system when used in combination with other immune-modulating remedies such as astragalus (*Astragalus membranaceus*) and echinacea (*Echinacea* spp.). Ginseng helps to enhance memory and recall and, combined with ginkgo (*Ginkgo biloba*), can be useful to the elderly as a preventative for dementia. With cancer-preventative activity, ginseng can be a helpful restorative when recovering from cancer (seek professional advice here). The root appears to help control blood sugar levels in diabetes, and it can relieve chronic or recurrent headaches when linked to overwork or exhaustion.

FRESH ROOT

men with low sperm count); to reduce menopausal fatigue and tiredness; to improve immune function and resistance to infection; and perhaps most importantly, to improve quality of life. Root and root extracts need to be of good quality for positive results and it is important to select a reputable brand or supplier; ideally, choose a standardized tincture or extract. Given the relatively high cost of ginseng root, adulterated products are not uncommon.

The root is harvested after four years; the older the root, the better its strength and quality.

ginseng extracts help to improve stamina

TABLETS

Butterbur

Petasites hybridus

Formerly used to treat plague, butterbur has long been used in Europe as a cough and cold remedy, and for stomach and gall bladder problems. Clinical trials suggest butterbur extract provides effective relief for migraines and hay fever, and the extract is now commonly available over the counter.

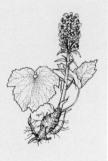

MEDICINAL USES

Part used Root

Key actions Anti-allergenic
● Anti-inflammatory ● Antispasmodic

Migraine, pain relief In clinical trials, butterbur extract reduced the frequency, duration, and intensity of migraine attacks. A safe treatment for migraines, the extract can be given to children as young as six years old, but only at the advised dosage. The extract may also help to relieve joint and menstrual pain.

Allergic rhinitis With its marked anti-allergenic activity, butterbur can bring allergic rhinitis, such as hay fever, under control. Butterbur can alleviate its troublesome symptoms such as nasal congestion, sore throat, and sneezing, especially if combined with an appropriate diet.

Coughs, colds, chest infections
Although not the first cough and cold remedy that comes to mind, butterbur extract can be useful in speeding up recovery from respiratory problems, such as chest coughs and bronchitis.

Gastrointestinal disorders Research suggests that butterbur reduces ulceration of the small intestine.

KEY INFORMATION

SAFETY	★ ★ ★ ★ ☆
TRADITIONAL USE	★ ★ ★ ⯪ ☆
RESEARCH	★ ★ ★ ★ ☆

BEST TAKEN AS Take only as a standardized extract (tablet) ✓ ✓ ✓
DOSAGE M (*see pp.44–45*)
CAUTIONS Do not take during pregnancy or while breast-feeding. Take only purified products where liver-toxic compounds have been removed. May rarely cause gastrointestinal upset or drowsiness. Restricted herb in some countries; not legally available in Australia. See also pp.42–51.

The wild plant, but not the extract, is toxic to the liver.

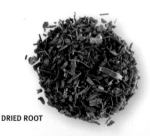

DRIED ROOT

Parsley

Petroselinum crispum

A useful food at any time, parsley is rich in a number of readily absorbable nutrients, including vitamin C and phytoestrogens, making it a valuable supplement, particularly during menopause. Medicinally, the root is preferred, having a distinct benefit on the urinary tract and in rheumatic problems.

MEDICINAL USES

Parts used Leaf • Root

Key actions Antirheumatic • Antispasmodic • Diuretic • Nutritive • Relieves gas • Stimulates menstruation

Menopausal symptoms, prevention of osteoporosis Moderately estrogenic, parsley leaf is a nutritious food supplement to take during menopause. Its relatively high boron content makes it a valuable supplement in natural approaches to preventing osteoporosis.

Urinary tract problems Commonly used with other urinary antiseptic remedies, parsley root can bring relief to the urinary tract in disorders such as mild cystitis and urethritis. It has traditionally been used in the prevention and treatment of kidney stones and is thought to aid the kidneys in the clearance of waste products that exacerbate muscle aches and stiffness.

Other uses Parsley has strong deodorizing properties and the leaf is commonly chewed to treat bad breath and to freshen the breath. It is said to mask the odor of garlic on the breath.

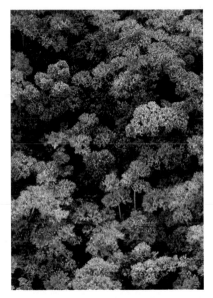

Parsley leaf is both flavoursome and rich in nutrients, notably significant levels of vitamins C and E, iron, boron, and phytoestrogens.

The root has a tonic activity on digestion, helping to relieve indigestion, gas, and bloating. Valued for its ability to promote menstrual blood flow, parsley at the recommended dosage can help in stimulating regular menstruation and relieving menstrual cramps. Parsley is thought to suppress breast milk production, so it is best avoided when breast-feeding. The root can be used to relieve arthritic symptoms.

DRIED LEAVES

KEY INFORMATION

SAFETY	★ ★ ★ ✰ ☆
TRADITIONAL USE	★ ★ ★ ★ ☆
RESEARCH	★ ★ ★ ☆ ☆
BEST TAKEN AS	Tincture ✓✓✓
DOSAGE	C (*see pp.44–45*)
OFTEN USED WITH	Meadowsweet (*Filipendula ulmaria*)
CAUTIONS	Do not use medicinally during pregnancy. See also pp.42–51.

Black catnip, Bahupatra

Phyllanthus amarus

A central Ayurvedic remedy for the liver, research into black catnip has produced conflicting results. Evidence suggests that it has liver-protective activity.

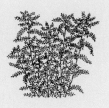

MEDICINAL USES

Part used Whole plant

Key actions Liver protector ● Lowers blood sugar levels ● Diuretic ● Antiviral

Liver disease Traditional use indicates that black catnip can help in disorders such as viral hepatitis, gall bladder disease, and gallstones. A safe remedy, it is best taken on professional advice.

Viral infections Following the herb's traditional use, black catnip makes a useful herb to combine with immune-modulating remedies such as echinacea (*Echinacea* spp.) in treating viral and other chronic infections.

LEAF

KEY INFORMATION

SAFETY	★ ★ ★ ★ ☆
TRADITIONAL USE	★ ★ ★ ★ ☆
RESEARCH	★ ★ ★ ☆ ☆

BEST TAKEN AS Decoction ✓✓✓ Tincture ✓✓ Tablet ✓
DOSAGE M, B (*see pp.44–45*)
CAUTIONS Rarely, may cause mild side effects. See also pp.42–51.

Pomegranate

Punica granatum

Recent research has focused on pomegranate juice as a preventative for prostate and colon cancer, and as a support for a healthy heart and circulation.

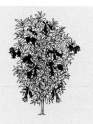

MEDICINAL USES

Part used Fruit

Key actions Antioxidant ● Antiviral ● Supports heart and circulation

KEY INFORMATION

SAFETY	★ ★ ★ ★ ★
TRADITIONAL USE	★ ★ ★ ☆ ☆
RESEARCH	★ ★ ★ ☆ ☆

BEST TAKEN AS Juice ✓✓✓
DOSAGE As food; M (*see pp.44–45*)
CAUTIONS Use fruit (seeds) or juice only; all other plant parts, including the rind, are toxic. See also pp.42–51.

Cancer preventative and cardio-vascular support With its very high levels of polyphenols, pomegranate juice clearly has powerful antioxidant activity. This makes the juice a valuable supplement to help prevent cancer development. The antioxidants also aid heart function and arterial health.

FRESH FRUIT

Other uses A traditional use of pomegranate juice (blended with seeds) is in the treatment of diarrhea.

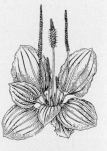

Plantain

Plantago major, P. lanceolata

Known in Gaelic as "the healing herb," plantain is a versatile herb that will benefit many conditions. Mostly used to support and strengthen mucous membranes throughout the body, plantain counters infection, reduces mucous membrane secretions, and supports tissue repair.

MEDICINAL USES

Part used Whole plant

Key actions Analgesic ● Anticatarrhal ● Antihemorrhagic ● Anti-inflammatory ● Antiviral ● Demulcent ● Wound healer

Congestion problems All congestion problems from ears to chest, and throughout the digestive tract, will benefit from plantain. It may be taken for colds, hay fever, sinusitis, cough, and sore throat. It is also treats acid indigestion, peptic ulcer, diarrhea, and irritable bowel. Best taken as tea, the tincture will also serve well. Take short-term for acute conditions, but long-term for chronic states such as sinus congestion, allergic rhinitis, and mucus colitis.

Broken or inflamed tissue An effective external application wherever tissue repair is needed, plantain also stimulates healing within the body, notably in the digestive and respiratory tracts.

Greater plantain (*P. major*) is preferred medicinally (*right*), but ribwort plantain (*P. lanceolata*) can be used in its place (*top left*).

ribwort plantain

FLOWERSPIKE   **DRIED LEAVES**

greater plantain is commonly used to heal wounds

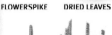

KEY INFORMATION

SAFETY	★ ★ ★ ★ ☆
TRADITIONAL USE	★ ★ ★ ★ ☆
RESEARCH	★ ★ ★ ☆ ☆

BEST TAKEN AS Infusion ✓✓✓
Tincture ✓✓
DOSAGE B (*see pp.44–45*)
OFTEN USED WITH Elderflower (*Sambucus nigra*)
CAUTIONS Rarely, may cause dermatitis. See also pp.42–51.

Cultivated since antiquity, the rose (*Rosa* spp.) is known as the "queen of flowers" for its beauty and fragrance. Rosewater distilled from the flowers is tonic to the skin.

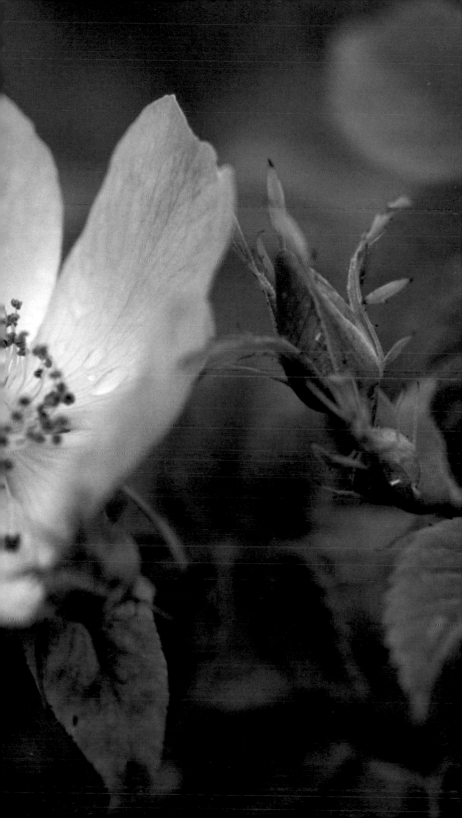

Rehmannia

Rehmannia glutinosa

A tonic for the liver and kidneys, rehmannia is also an important anti-inflammatory herb. In its native China, it is used to cool fever in chronic illnesses.

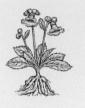

MEDICINAL USES

Part used Root

Key actions Adrenal tonic ● Anti-hemorrhagic ● Anti-inflammatory ● Reduces fever

Chronic inflammation A key herb used to control inflammation in chronic inflammatory disorders, such as rheumatoid arthritis and polymyalgia rheumatica (especially where exhaustion and weakness are factors), rehmannia is best taken on professional advice.

FLOWERS AND LEAVES

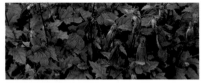

KEY INFORMATION

SAFETY	★★★★⯪
TRADITIONAL USE	★★★★☆
RESEARCH	★★★☆☆

BEST TAKEN AS Tincture ✓✓✓ Decoction ✓✓
DOSAGE B (*see pp.44–45*)
CAUTIONS During pregnancy, take only after consulting a professional. Can occasionally cause diarrhea. See also pp.42–51.

Rose

Rosa spp.

Rosewater, distilled from the petals, soothes and tones the skin. A syrup from the hips of the dog rose (*R. canina*) is given to children to improve resistance to infection.

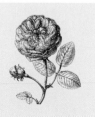

MEDICINAL USES

Part used Petals ● Fruit (hips)

Key actions Anti-inflammatory ● Astringent ● Tonic

KEY INFORMATION

SAFETY	★★★★★
TRADITIONAL USE	★★★★★
RESEARCH	★★⯪☆☆

BEST TAKEN AS Syrup ✓✓✓ Aromatic water (topically) ✓✓✓
DOSAGE C (*see pp.44–45*)
CAUTIONS Rarely, fruit or syrup may cause gastrointestinal upset. See also pp.42–51.

Skin toner Rosewater makes a valued application for lax tissue, including burns, mouth ulcers, chapped hands, and sore eyes.

petals are tonic and astringent

FLOWER

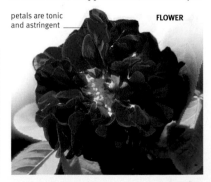

Rhubarb

Rheum officinalis

A well-tolerated and moderately powerful laxative, rhubarb exerts a positive influence on the liver, gallbladder, and intestines. At a low dose, its astringent actions predominate to control diarrhea, while at normal dose, it acts as an irritant laxative.

MEDICINAL USES

Part used Root

Key actions Antibacterial ● Astringent ● Bitter ● Blood cleanser ● Laxative

Constipation Rhubarb root is best used as a short-term remedy for constipation when other approaches, such as increased fiber in the diet or linseed, fail. Take two 0.5g capsules with chamomile or ginger tea in the evening. Repeat for up to two weeks. If the problem persists, seek professional advice.

Other uses In combination with other remedies, rhubarb has significant therapeutic use in gastrointestinal infection and chronic inflammation such as Crohn's disease.

KEY INFORMATION

SAFETY	★ ★ ★ ★ ☆
TRADITIONAL USE	★ ★ ★ ★ ☆
RESEARCH	★ ★ ★ ★ ☆

BEST TAKEN AS Capsule ✓✓✓ Tincture ✓✓

DOSAGE C (*see pp.44–45*)

OFTEN USED WITH Ginger (*Zingiber officinalis*)

CAUTIONS Do not take during pregnancy or while breast-feeding. Do not give to children. May cause gastrointestinal upset. See also pp.42–51.

root is an effective laxative

POWDERED ROOT

Rhubarb root has mild antimicrobial activity against a range of bacteria, fungi, and viruses.

Golden root, Arctic root

Rhodiola rosea

Found in mountainous regions and tundra as far north as the Arctic, golden root has benefits similar in many ways to ginseng. A key remedy for long-term stress and physical and mental fatigue, it supports the body's stress response.

MEDICINAL USES

Part used Root

Key actions Adaptogen
- Anti-inflammatory
- Antioxidant ● Protects heart
- Tonic for males

Physical endurance and long-term stress An important endurance herb, golden root helps the body and mind adapt efficiently to increased physical and mental demands, as in sports training or studying for exams. It also improves work performance. It can be valuable in depleted states such as chronic fatigue and nervous exhaustion, although care should be taken to start at a low dose and increase it slowly.

Golden root can be taken to prevent altitude sickness.

KEY INFORMATION

SAFETY   ★ ★ ★ ★ ☆
TRADITIONAL USE   ★ ★ ★ ★ ☆
RESEARCH   ★ ★ ★ ★ ☆
BEST TAKEN AS Standardized extract (rosavin): Tablet, tincture ✓✓✓
DOSAGE M (*see pp.44–45*)
OFTEN USED WITH Ginseng (*Panax ginseng*)
CAUTION Can cause irritability and sleep disturbance. Not advisable in manic and bipolar disorders. See also pp.42–51.

root extract relieves stress

FRESH ROOT   **TABLETS**

Depressive mood Though golden root does not as yet have established antidepressant activity, it does appear to help raise mood and vitality in those who have a tendency to suffer from depression.

Blackcurrant

Ribes nigrum

The tart, crisp flavor of blackcurrant reflects the fruit's high vitamin C content and marked antioxidant activity. Long given to children to protect them from colds and throat infection, the fruit, juice, and extracts are thought to have significant anti-inflammatory and antiviral activity.

MEDICINAL USES

Parts used Bud • Fruit • Leaf • Seed oil

Key actions Adrenal support (buds) • Anti-inflammatory • Antioxidant • Astringent • Diuretic (leaves)

Immune support Following traditional use, blackcurrant juice or extract can be taken regularly to maintain healthy resistance to viral infection, including colds, flu, and herpes sores. It is likely to speed recovery from infection as well. Avoid sweetened concentrates.

Allergy and chronic inflammation

In France, the buds are thought to support adrenal gland function and are prescribed to treat allergic and inflammatory conditions such as asthma. The seed oil, which possesses high levels of omega-6 essential fatty acids (GLA) with similar properties to evening primrose oil, can be taken

FRESH LEAF

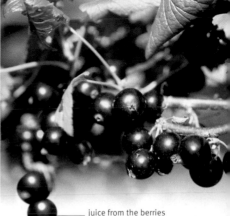

juice from the berries can relieve indigestion

Blackcurrant is grown mainly in eastern Europe for its sour-sweet fruit. The leaves and berries are harvested in early and late summer respectively.

to control inflammation in conditions such as rheumatoid arthritis and multiple sclerosis.

Circulatory tonic With their high levels of antioxidant anthocyanins, the fruit and leaves can be taken long-term as a treatment to strengthen the circulation, including the capillaries. The juice or extract can be taken daily for several months to help improve circulatory problems, such as capillary fragility and varicose veins.

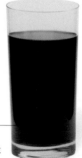

juice is high in vitamin C and antioxidants

BLACKCURRANT JUICE

KEY INFORMATION

SAFETY	★ ★ ★ ★ ★
TRADITIONAL USE	★ ★ ★ ★ ☆
RESEARCH	★ ★ ★ ☆ ☆

BEST TAKEN AS Juice/extract ✓✓✓ Infusion ✓✓ Seed oil ✓

DOSAGE As recommended

CAUTIONS None known. See also pp.42–51.

A Mediterranean herb, rosemary (*Rosmarinus officinalis*) symbolizes fidelity between lovers, an association that may have been made on account of its ability to improve memory.

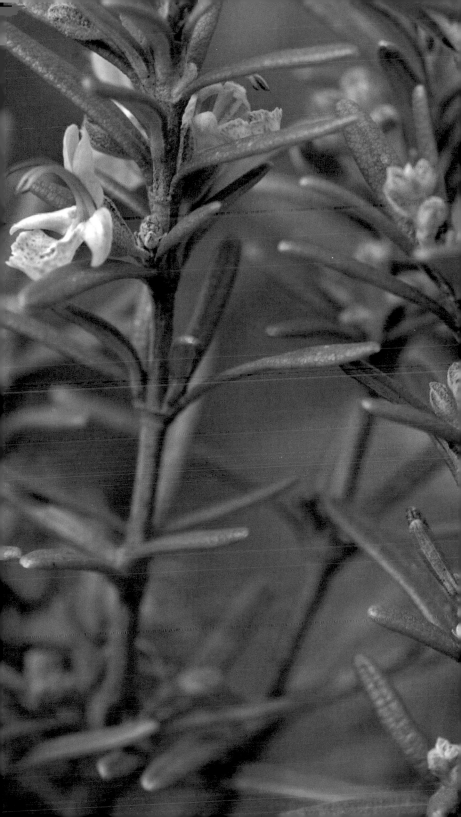

Rosemary

Rosmarinus officinalis

Few herbs are as well known as rosemary, especially for its distinctive aroma. Traditionally used to strengthen memory and recall, it is frequently taken to aid study and exam performance, and to ward off mental exhaustion.

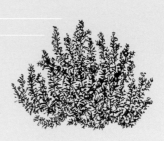

MEDICINAL USES

Parts used Leaf ● Essential oil

Key actions Anti-inflammatory ● Antioxidant ● Antispasmodic ● Circulatory stimulant ● Digestive tonic ● Nerve tonic

Headache, migraine, nervous exhaustion An infusion of rosemary can bring quick relief to headaches caused by overwork and nervous tension. For headaches linked to high blood pressure, combine with lindenflowers (*Tilia* spp.). It can also prove helpful in migraine.

Digestion, poor circulation, low energy Tonic and antioxidant, rosemary stimulates digestion and blood flow throughout the body, proving helpful for those with low energy levels, especially where linked to low blood pressure or poor appetite.

KEY INFORMATION

SAFETY	★ ★ ★ ★ ☆
TRADITIONAL USE	★ ★ ★ ★ ☆
RESEARCH	★ ★ ★ ☆ ☆

BEST TAKEN AS Infusion ✓✓✓ Tincture ✓✓ Essential oil (topically) at maximum 5% dilution in carrier oil ✓
DOSAGE C (*see pp.44–45*)
OFTEN USED WITH Lavender (*Lavandula officinalis*)
CAUTIONS Rarely, may cause contact allergy. See also pp.42–51.

It is a key herb for those failing to thrive, either after long-term illness or where digestion and circulation are weak. For best results, take rosemary tea or tincture before meals for several months.

aromatic leaves contain essential oil

Hair tonic An infusion made from the leaves acts as a natural hair conditioner, toning the scalp and strengthening the hair.

leaves are used to relieve headaches and tension

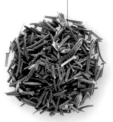

DRIED LEAVES

Rosemary tea or diluted essential oil makes an excellent rub for sore and aching muscles and joints.

Raspberry

Rubus ideaus

Known in classical times as an aid to childbirth, raspberry leaf is thought to act on the womb, relaxing the cervix, and toning the muscles that contract during labor. Recent studies indicate that it is a safe remedy that shortens labor and reduces the likelihood of a forceps delivery.

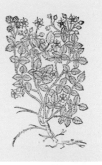

MEDICINAL USES

Part used Leaf

Key actions Aids preparation for childbirth ● Antidiarrheal ● Astringent

To aid preparation for childbirth Take raspberry leaf as an infusion or capsule on a daily basis for the last three months of pregnancy, and freely during labor to ease contractions. The normal daily dose is 1–2 cups of tea.

FRESH LEAF

DRIED LEAVES
leaves make an effective gargle for sore throat

KEY INFORMATION

SAFETY	★ ★ ★ ★ ☆
TRADITIONAL USE	★ ★ ★ ★ ☆
RESEARCH	★ ★ ★ ☆ ☆

BEST TAKEN AS Infusion ✓✓✓ Capsule ✓✓ Tablet ✓
DOSAGE B (*see pp.44–45*)
CAUTIONS Do not take during first 3 months of pregnancy. During last 3 months, best taken after consulting an herbal or medical practitioner. See also pp.42–51.

Heavy menstrual bleeding Raspberry leaf can help control heavy menstrual bleeding, combining well with yarrow (*Achillea millefolium*) to reduce blood loss. It is sometimes taken to relieve premenstrual symptoms and period pains.

Other uses With its strong astringent action, an infusion of the leaves makes a gentle-acting and effective remedy for diarrhea and loose bowel movements in children. It is equally useful as a gargle for sore throats and a lotion for sore eyes.

Raspberry is grown mostly for its delicious-tasting fruit, which can be made into a syrup or vinegar; traditionally, it was used to treat feverish states.

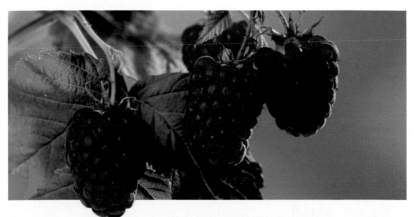

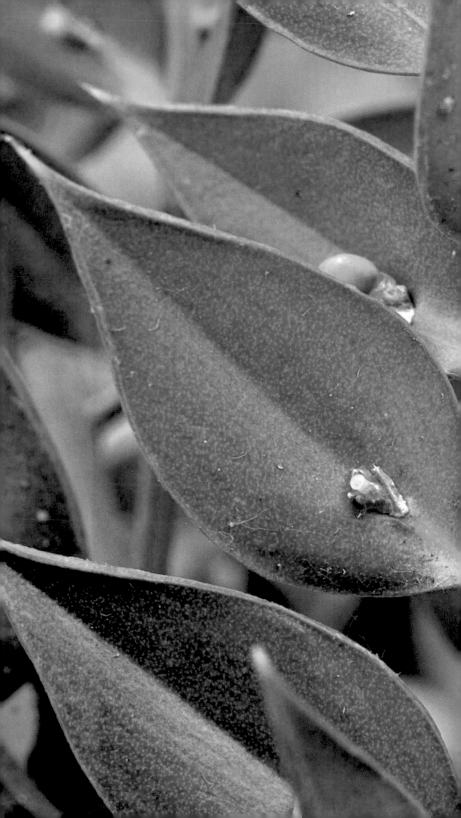

A venous tonic, butcher's broom (*Ruscus aculeatus*) has leaf-like leathery branches with a terminal spine. Traditionally, it was used as a diuretic and to treat kidney disorders.

Sheep's sorrel

Rumex acetosella

A small dock-type plant, sheep's sorrell is rarely used as a medicine on its own. Its chief therapeutic use lies in its role as the principal remedy in the Essiac formula.

MEDICINAL USES

Part used Whole plant

Key actions Anti-inflammatory
• Diuretic • Laxative

Claimed cancer cure The Essiac formula (a cancer treatment devised in the 1920s by the Canadian nurse Rene Caisse, following a native Ojibwa recipe) comprises sheep's sorrel, burdock (*Arctium lappa*), slippery elm (*Ulmus rubra*), and rhubarb (*Rhubarb officinalis*). No detailed investigation has yet taken place into its clinical effects. Burdock (*Arctium lappa*) and rhubarb (*Rhubarb officinalis*), but not sheep's sorrel, are known to possess anticancer activity, and prepared Essiac tea has strong antioxidant properties.

AERIAL PARTS

KEY INFORMATION

SAFETY	★ ★½ ☆ ☆
TRADITIONAL USE	★ ★½ ☆ ☆
RESEARCH	★ ½ ☆ ☆ ☆
BEST TAKEN AS	Infusion ✓✓✓
Tincture ✓✓	
DOSAGE	T, C (see pp.44–45)

CAUTIONS Do not take excess doses of root. Do not give to children. Take only after consulting a physician. May occasionally cause gastrointestinal upset or skin reactions. See also pp.42–51.

Butcher's broom

Ruscus aculeatus

An unusual-looking native European plant with stiff spiky "leaves," butcher's broom has been investigated in detail as a remedy for problems affecting the veins.

MEDICINAL USES

Part used Root

Key actions Anti-inflammatory
• Laxative • Venous tonic

KEY INFORMATION

SAFETY	★ ★ ★ ★ ½
TRADITIONAL USE	★ ★ ★ ½ ☆
RESEARCH	★ ★ ★ ★ ☆
BEST TAKEN AS	Capsule ✓✓✓ Tablet ✓✓✓
Tincture ✓	
DOSAGE	M (see pp.44–45)

CAUTIONS May occasionally cause gastrointestinal upset. See also pp.42–51.

Venous insufficiency Butcher's broom contracts vein walls, leading to reduced fluid loss into surrounding areas. It may need to be taken long-term for varicosed leg veins and to reverse fluid retention in the lower legs. Unlike horse chestnut (*Aesculus hippocastanum*), it has little positive effect on the arteries.

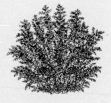

root aids venous problems

FRESH ROOT

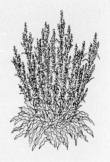

Yellow dock

Rumex crispus

A common weed and wayside plant, yellow dock has a deep taproot that draws up iron and other minerals from the soil, presenting them in an accessible form for absorption. The root is therefore prescribed in cases of iron-deficiency anemia, although its main use is for sluggish bowels and mild constipation.

MEDICINAL USES

Parts used Root ● Leaf (topically)

Key actions Detoxifier ● Laxative

Chronic skin problems Yellow dock is best used in combination with other herbs rather than on its own. It fits well in formulas that contain other "blood cleansers" such as burdock *(Arctium lappa)* to support bowel clearance and liver detoxification. Yellow dock is called for in conditions involving chronic toxicity, including skin disorders such as acne and boils, eczema, and psoriasis. Often the best approach is to take small amounts regularly over several months, promoting gradual but effective detoxification. Other types of chronic illness that involve poor elimination, like swollen glands and throat infection, can also benefit from the root's cleansing activity.

Other uses Yellow dock combines well with nettle *(Urtica dioica)* in allergic and rheumatic conditions. Both herbs also contain appreciable levels of iron and can be used as a natural iron supplement in mild cases of anemia.

KEY INFORMATION

SAFETY	★ ★ ★ ★ ☆
TRADITIONAL USE	★ ★ ★ ★ ☆
RESEARCH	★ ☆ ☆ ☆ ☆

BEST TAKEN AS Tincture ✓✓✓
Decoction ✓✓
DOSAGE C *(see pp.44–45)*
OFTEN USED WITH Burdock *(Arctium lappa)*
CAUTIONS Do not take excess doses of root. Do not take leaves internally. Not advisable during pregnancy. See also pp.42–51.

Yellow dock is a traditional remedy for nettle stings; rub the fresh leaves firmly onto the affected area. Do not take the leaves internally, as they are poisonous.

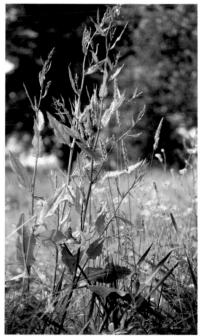

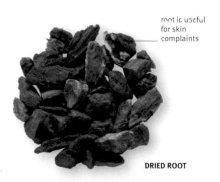

root is useful for skin complaints

DRIED ROOT

Willow bark, White willow

Salix alba

An ancient remedy for aches and pains, fevers, and rheumatic conditions, willow bark contains aspirin-like substances. It is often thought of as the herbal equivalent of aspirin, but its mode of action is only partly the same—it cannot be used as a straightforward aspirin replacement.

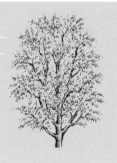

MEDICINAL USES

Part used Bark

Key actions Analgesic ● Anti-inflammatory ● Astringent ● Relieves fever

Aches and pains The bark may be taken as a first aid remedy for headaches, toothaches, and back pain. Its main use is in muscle and joint inflammation, pain and stiffness, and for conditions such as sports injuries and gout. The herb causes few side effects and may be preferable to aspirin-type anti-inflammatories in conditions such as osteoarthritis that require long-term use.

Fever Take an infusion (perhaps with ginger, *Zingiber officinalis*) to control fevers and to relieve the malaise and discomfort that accompanies acute infection. If the temperature is 102.2°F (39°C) or above, seek professional advice immediately.

KEY INFORMATION

SAFETY	★★★★☆
TRADITIONAL USE	★★★★★
RESEARCH	★★★⯪☆

BEST TAKEN AS Tincture ✓✓✓ Capsule ✓✓ Infusion ✓

DOSAGE A (*see pp.44–45*)

OFTEN USED WITH Devil's claw (*Harpagophytum procumbens*)

CAUTIONS Do not take if allergic to aspirin, or while breast-feeding. Do not give to children with viral infections. Can cause allergic reactions. May occasionally cause gastrointestinal upset. See also pp.42–51.

bark relieves stiffness

FRESH BARK

Native to much of Europe, willow bark thrives in damp areas and on river banks. It is thought to treat "damp" conditions within the body.

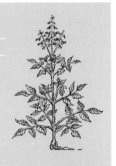

Dan shen, Asian red sage

Salvia miltiorrhiza

A cousin of garden sage, dan shen is *the* Chinese remedy for heart and circulation, and has been used for over 2,000 years. The root has an impressive range of activity on the cardiovascular system, benefiting conditions such as high blood pressure, poor peripheral circulation, and heart failure.

MEDICINAL USES

Part used Root

Key actions Anticoagulant ● Lowers blood pressure ● Sedative ● Tonic for heart and circulation

Heart tonic Similar in some respects to hawthorn (*Crataegus* spp.), dan shen increases blood flow through the coronary arteries and has a marked relaxant action on the circulation to the heart, making it a key remedy for angina and a weak or under-performing heart. Dan shen is best taken on the recommendation of an herbal or medical practitioner.

High blood pressure and poor peripheral circulation Dan shen relaxes arterial circulation and thins the blood, both factors that contribute to a lower blood pressure and stronger circulation to the hands and feet.

Other uses The herb has strong anticoagulant activity—seek professional advice if taking blood-thinning medication or where a tendency toward bleeding or bruising exists.

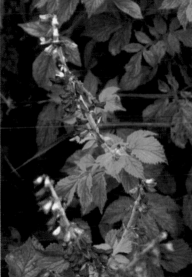

A native Chinese herb, dan shen is cultivated in northeastern China and Inner Mongolia, and sold in herbal markets across China as a circulatory stimulant.

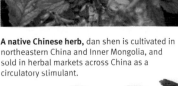

DRIED CHOPPED ROOT

root has strong anticoagulant activity

tincture is taken to relieve angina

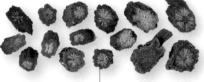

TINCTURE

KEY INFORMATION

SAFETY	★ ★ ★ ☆ ☆
TRADITIONAL USE	★ ★ ★ ★ ☆
RESEARCH	★ ★ ★ ☆ ☆

BEST TAKEN AS Decoction ✓✓✓ Tincture ✓✓ Tablet ✓

DOSAGE C (*see pp.44–45*)

CAUTIONS Do not take during pregnancy. Do not take with prescribed blood-thinning medication. May occasionally cause gastrointestinal upset. See also pp.42–51.

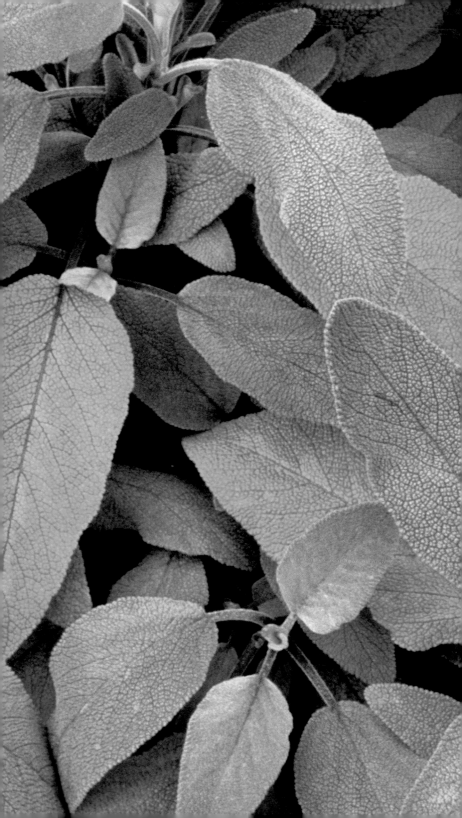

The bluish-purple flowers of sage (*Salvia officinalis*) make a sharp contrast to its gray-green leaves. The Latin name *Salvia* means "to cure," echoing the medieval perception of the herb.

Sage, Spanish sage

Salvia officinalis, S. lavandulifolia

In 1551, the English herbalist William Turner noted that sage "restores natural heat ... comforts the vital spirits ... helps the memory, and quickens the senses." Such praise is not misplaced for sage, which is truly a versatile and effective tonic.

MEDICINAL USES

Part used Leaf

Key actions Antimicrobial
- Antioxidant ● Astringent
- Digestive tonic ● Estrogenic
- General tonic ● Reduces sweating

Mouth ulcers, sore throat, excess catarrh With its valuable astringent properties, sage counters infections, such as mouth ulcers and sore throat, and dries up catarrh. The infusion makes an excellent mouthwash and gargle for local infections. Sage combines well with herbs such as echinacea (*Echinacea* spp.) for recurrent problems.

DRIED LEAVES

Despite its medicinal value, sage is most commonly known as a culinary herb.

fresh leaf is a first aid remedy for insect bites

Menopausal symptoms Cold sage tea sipped in small doses through the day is a traditional remedy for menopausal symptoms such as sweating, hot flashes, and headache.

Poor memory, stress, and anxiety Recent research points to sage as a potential remedy for early stages of dementia. Its tranquillizing properties help relieve stress and anxiety, and also improve mental vitality and memory. Spanish sage is preferable for long-term use—its low thujone content makes it safer than ordinary sage.

SAGE TINCTURE

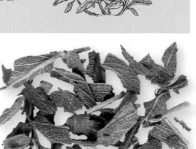

KEY INFORMATION

SAFETY	★ ★ ★ ⯪ ☆
TRADITIONAL USE	★ ★ ★ ★ ⯪
RESEARCH	★ ★ ★ ☆ ☆

BEST TAKEN AS Infusion ✓✓✓ Tincture ✓✓ Capsule ✓
DOSAGE C (*see pp.44–45*)
OFTEN USED WITH Alfalfa (*Medicago sativa*)
CAUTIONS Do not take during pregnancy and while breast-feeding. Excessive doses can be toxic. See also pp.42–51.

Schisandra, Wu wei zi

Schisandra chinensis

Known in China as "the five-flavored herb" for the distinctively sour and slightly salty flavor of its berries, schisandra has been traditionally used as a sexual tonic for both men and women. The herb is thought to tone the kidneys and sexual organs, protect the liver, and improve mental stamina.

MEDICINAL USES

Part used Fruit

Key actions Adaptogen ● Antioxidant ● Mild antidepressant ● Protects liver ● Tonic

Reduced vitality A few schisandra berries chewed every day will increase physical and mental vitality and help combat stress. Schisandra is often combined with ginkgo (*Ginkgo biloba*) to boost memory and improve concentration. With its mild sedative and antidepressant qualities, schisandra can help with depressive states linked to long-term stress and mental exhaustion. Schisandra can add zest to life and for this reason can be a valuable tonic where libido is low.

Liver disorders Schisandra improves liver health and aids in the effective metabolism of toxins. Chronic liver disorders in general can benefit, including chronic viral hepatitis. In this situation, take the herb only with professional recommendation.

Other uses Schisandra is used in the treatment of respiratory infections such as chronic cough, shortness of breath, and wheezing. It may also be used to

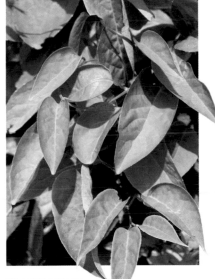

It is said that if taken for 100 days, schisandra purifies the blood and brightens the mind.

treat diarrhea and dysentery, failing eyesight and hearing, as well as skin problems such as urticaria and eczema.

DRIED FRUIT

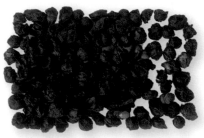

KEY INFORMATION

SAFETY	★★★★☆
TRADITIONAL USE	★★★★★
RESEARCH	★★★☆☆

BEST TAKEN AS Dried fruit or powder ✓✓✓ Tincture ✓✓
DOSAGE C (*see pp.44–45*)
OFTEN USED WITH Astragalus (*Astragalus chinensis*)
CAUTIONS Do not take during pregnancy. Can cause mild digestive irritation. See also pp.42–51.

Elder

Sambucus nigra

Although poorly researched, elder is a safe and effective domestic remedy for ear, nose, and throat problems, whose traditional use in Europe goes back to pre-classical times. The creamy white flowers are often collected to make wine, but the tincture or hot infusion are therapeutically more effective.

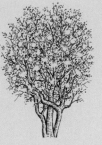

MEDICINAL USES

Parts used Flower • Fruit

Key actions Anticatarrhal • Anti-inflammatory • Antioxidant • Antiviral • Diaphoretic (stimulates sweating)

Common cold, flu, and fever

Elderflowers make an excellent cooling infusion for cold symptoms, flu-like colds, and mild feverish states by easing symptoms as well as countering infection. They combine well with yarrow (*Achillea millefolium*). Drink the infusion hot, sweetened with honey. Ripe elderberries contain high levels of vitamin C, and contain strong antioxidants. Take elderberry syrup or extract to counter infection and speed recovery. A recent clinical trial found that elderberry extract shortened recovery time in people

KEY INFORMATION

SAFETY	★ ★ ★ ★ ☆
TRADITIONAL USE	★ ★ ★ ★ ☆
RESEARCH	★ ★ ☆ ☆ ☆

BEST TAKEN AS Flower: Infusion, tincture ✓✓✓ Fruit: Tincture, extract ✓✓✓
DOSAGE A (*see pp.44–45*)
OFTEN USED WITH Yarrow (*Achillea millefolium*)
CAUTIONS None known. Do not consume unripe berries. See also pp.42–51.

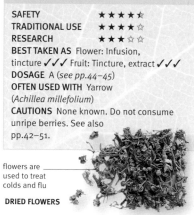

flowers are used to treat colds and flu

DRIED FLOWERS

suffering from influenza. In either form, the berries can be taken to improve resistance to infection and reduce a tendency toward recurring colds, sore throats, and coughs. Elderberry extract is available as an over-the-counter remedy, and can safely be given to children.

Congestive problems of ear, nose, and throat

Elderflowers can dry and tone mucous membranes lining the nose and throat, reducing sneezing, itchiness, and a "runny nose" in conditions such as allergic rhinitis and hay fever. Combining elderflowers with nettle (*Urtica dioica*) is more effective in such cases. Elderflowers are often used in chronic catarrhal problems affecting the sinuses and the middle ear. In combination with other remedies, the flowers are also useful in treating chest infections such as bronchitis and pleurisy.

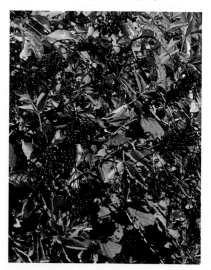

Found in temperate regions all over the world and often cultivated, the elder tree is native to Europe and thrives in woods, hedges, and on waste ground.

NATURE'S CURE-ALL

"If the medicinal properties of its leaves, bark, and berries were fully known, I cannot tell what our countryman could ail for which he might not fetch a remedy from every hedge, either for sickness, or wounds. The buds boiled in water gruel have effected wonders in a fever; the spring buds are excellently wholesome in pattages; and small ale in which Elder flowers have been infused is esteemed by many...." John Evelyn, 1664.

FLOWER CLUSTER

The Elder tree is traditionally known as "nature's medicine chest." The berries make excellent wines and winter cordials that relieve colds.

Other uses Elderflower tea, taken hot rather than cold, is thought to act as a diuretic, stimulating urine flow. It is traditionally taken to relieve rheumatic aches and pains. A cold elderflower infusion can be used as a wash for sore and inflamed eyes, including conjunctivitis. Mildly astringent, it is believed to relieve skin conditions such as acne, eczema, and psoriasis.

Baical skullcap

Scutellaria baicalensis

Used in both Chinese and Japanese herbal medicine, baical skullcap is a major remedy for allergic and inflammatory states. In traditional terms, it clears "hot and damp" conditions such as fever and dysentery; in the West it is mainly used to treat asthma, hay fever, and allergies.

MEDICINAL USES

Part used Root

Key actions Anti-allergenic ● Antibacterial ● Anti-inflammatory

Allergies The herb can reduce the intensity of allergic reactions (usually in combination with other remedies) such as asthma, eczema, hay fever, and nettle rash. Best results are likely to occur when taken on professional advice.

Gastrointestinal problems
A useful remedy for diarrhea and gastrointestinal infection, baical skullcap is also helpful in upper digestive problems such as nausea and vomiting.

FRESH ROOT

root has anti-inflammatory properties

Other uses In China, the herb is used for respiratory infection, including colds, cough, and bronchitis, and figures in many prescriptions for high blood pressure. It appears to have anticancer properties and a *kampo* (traditional Japanese system of medicine) formula containing the herb is prescribed to support immune function in cancer. In the West, baical skullcap is prescribed for high blood pressure and chronic inflammatory diseases such as rheumatoid arthritis.

A decoction made from the root can relieve chest colds and wheezing.

TINCTURE

KEY INFORMATION

SAFETY	★ ★ ★ ★ ☆
TRADITIONAL USE	★ ★ ★ ★ ☆
RESEARCH	★ ★ ★ ☆ ☆

BEST TAKEN AS Tincture ✓✓✓ Capsule ✓✓ Decoction ✓
DOSAGE B (*see pp.44–45*)
CAUTIONS Very rarely, may cause side effects. See also pp.42–51.

Skullcap

Scutellaria lateriflora

A key nerve tonic, skullcap is thought to have a "deeper" action on the nervous system than almost any other herb. Although poorly researched, it is used as a standard remedy for anxiety and nervous exhaustion, as well as related symptoms such as disturbed sleep, lowered mood, and headache.

MEDICINAL USES

Parts used Aerial parts

Key actions Antispasmodic • Mild bitter • Nerve tonic • Sedative

Nervous tension and anxiety Skullcap is used primarily as a nerve tonic and a restorative. Taken on its own or in combination with other herbs, it soothes a tense and tired nervous system, and is helpful for headaches and migraine, an inability to relax and poor sleep. Considered a "food" for the nervous system, skullcap often proves helpful in conditions where nervous debility is a factor, whether as the result of long-term stress, insomnia, or chronic pain. A range of other nerve-related disorders such as shock, dizziness, tinnitus, and chronic fatigue may also benefit. The herb's antispasmodic action makes it useful in relieving the taut and tensed muscles that so often accompany anxiety and worry. Skullcap is included in many over-the-counter herbal formulations for anxiety and sleep problems.

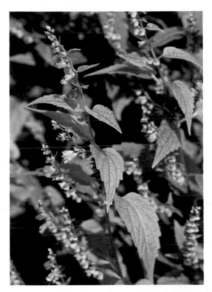

Easily recognizable by its distinctive seed capsules and pink to blue flowers, skullcap is a native of the USA and Canada.

aerial parts are used in preparations to aid sleep

DRIED AERIAL PARTS

Premenstrual syndrome (PMS) Usually combined with chaste berry (*Vitex agnus-castus*) and taken in small doses throughout the menstrual cycle, skullcap can take the edge off symptoms of PMS such as oversensitivity, nervous irritability, and breast pain and tenderness. It may also relieve menstrual cramps.

KEY INFORMATION

SAFETY	★ ★ ★ ★ ☆
TRADITIONAL USE	★ ★ ★ ★ ☆
RESEARCH	★ ☆ ☆ ☆ ☆

BEST TAKEN AS Tincture ✓✓✓
Capsule ✓✓ Tablet ✓
DOSAGE C (*see pp.44–45*)
OFTEN USED WITH Valerian (*Valeriana officinalis*)
CAUTIONS None known at normal dosage.
See also pp.42–51.

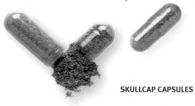

SKULLCAP CAPSULES

Saw palmetto

Serenoa repens

In many European countries, saw palmetto is used as a standard medical treatment for enlarged prostate gland. Strong research evidence supports its use in treating benign prostatic hypertrophy (BPH) and the urinary difficulties that go with it.

MEDICINAL USES

Part used Fruit

Key actions Anti-inflammatory
● Prostate remedy ● Male tonic

Prostate gland and urinary tract problems Best taken as a standardized extract, saw palmetto will often prove effective in relieving mild to moderate BPH symptoms, improving urine flow and effective emptying of the bladder. A useful anti-inflammatory, it can also

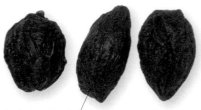

berries have diuretic and tonic activity

DRIED BERRIES

be taken to treat an inflamed prostate (prostatitis) and has longstanding traditional use in chronic urinary tract problems such as cystitis and urethritis.

Sexual tonic Saw palmetto is commonly regarded as an aphrodisiac and male sexual tonic. It undoubtedly has hormonal activity and may improve libido in both men and women.

Polycystic ovary syndrome The extract is thought to have anti-androgenic activity and is used to treat polycystic ovary syndrome, a gynecological condition in which androgen levels are raised.

A small palm tree native to Florida and the Gulf of Mexico, saw palmetto grows in sand dunes along the coast.

KEY INFORMATION

SAFETY	★★★★☆
TRADITIONAL USE	★★★★☆
RESEARCH	★★★★☆

BEST TAKEN AS Standardized extract ✓✓✓
DOSAGE C (*see pp.44–45*)
OFTEN USED WITH Nettle root (*Urtica dioica*)
CAUTIONS Occasionally may cause gastrointestinal upset, headache, or dizziness. See also pp.42–51.

Milk thistle

Silybum marianum syn. *Carduus marianus*

Extensively researched over the last 30 years, milk thistle is a powerful friend of the liver that protects against poisoning, toxicity, and inflammatory damage. It stimulates liver repair and regeneration, inhibits inflammatory processes resulting from infection, and promotes effective liver detoxification.

MEDICINAL USES

Part used Seed

Key actions Antioxidant ● Protects liver ● Stimulates breast milk

Liver disorders Best taken as a standardized extract, milk thistle helps to maintain a healthy liver. It can be taken whenever the liver is under stress, which is usually reflected in raised liver enzyme levels. The seeds contain silymarin, a substance that protects the liver against poisoning, the most dramatic instance of this being the herb's established ability to prevent poisoning where death cap mushrooms have been eaten. Medical conditions that can respond well to milk thistle include

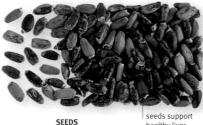

SEEDS

seeds support healthy liver function

raised cholesterol levels, acute and chronic viral hepatitis, chronic liver disease, and alcohol-induced liver cirrhosis. In liver disease and when taken to protect liver function during chemotherapy, use only on professional advice. Long-term use of milk thistle appears to be safe.

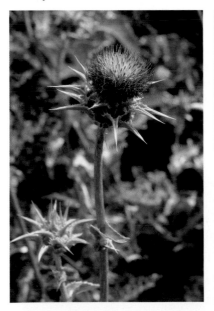

KEY INFORMATION

SAFETY	★ ★ ★ ★ ☆
TRADITIONAL USE	★ ★ ★ ★ ★
RESEARCH	★ ★ ★ ★ ☆

BEST TAKEN AS Standardized extract (standardized to 140mg silymarin) ✓✓✓
DOSAGE M, B (*see pp.44–45*)
CAUTIONS May occasionally cause gastrointestinal upset and allergic reactions. See also pp.42–51.

CAPSULE

Other uses As its name implies, the seeds were taken by nursing mothers to improve the supply of breast milk, a use that remains as applicable today as in the past. It has a persistent reputation as a remedy for depressed mood.

Native to the Mediterranean, milk thistle grows in the wild throughout Europe. It thrives mainly on waste ground, but is also cultivated as an ornamental plant.

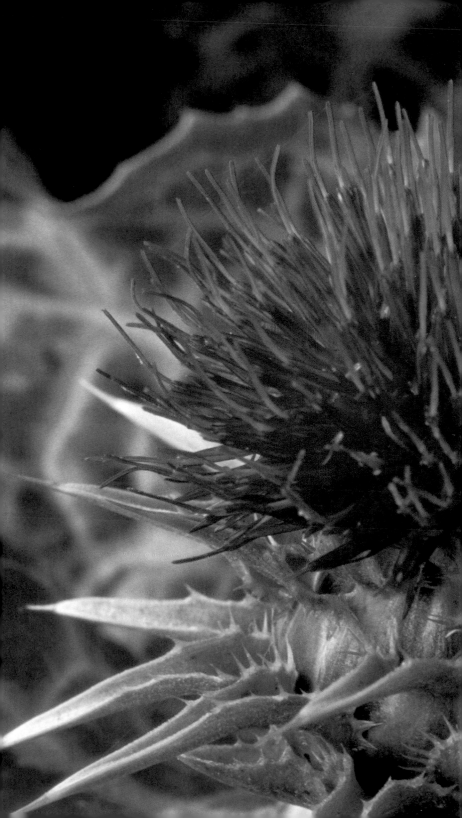

A European herb, milk thistle (*Silybum marianus*) has white markings on its leaves caused, folklore has it, by the Virgin Mary's milk. It is today the main herbal remedy for liver problems.

Sarsaparilla

Smilax spp.

Long used in the Americas and Europe, sarsaparilla is a valuable remedy for chronic infections, chronic inflammatory disease, and menopausal problems.

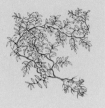

MEDICINAL USES

Part used Root

Key actions Anti-inflammatory ● Anti-rheumatic ● Detoxicant ● Diuretic ● Tonic

Skin disorders Sarsaparilla is used to treat psoriasis and eczema, particularly where itchiness is a major factor. It is best taken in combination, for example with yellow dock (*Rumex crispus*).

Menopausal problems Sarsaparilla can help with menopausal problems linked with skin or arthritic symptoms.

FRESH LEAVES

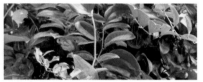

KEY INFORMATION

SAFETY   ★ ★ ★ ★ ☆
TRADITIONAL USE   ★ ★ ★ ★ ☆
RESEARCH   ★ ★ ☆ ☆ ☆
BEST TAKEN AS Decoction ✓✓✓
Tincture ✓✓
DOSAGE C (*see pp.44–45*)
CAUTIONS High doses may cause side effects. Seek professional advice if taking prescribed medication. See also pp.42–51.

Betony

Stachys officinalis

Although poorly researched, betony has a wealth of traditional uses, with one classical writer recommending it for as many as 47 illnesses.

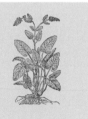

MEDICINAL USES

Parts used Aerial parts

Key actions Astringent ● Mild bitter ● Mild sedative ● Nerve tonic

KEY INFORMATION

SAFETY   ★ ★ ★ ★ ☆
TRADITIONAL USE   ★ ★ ★ ☆ ☆
RESEARCH   ★ ☆ ☆ ☆ ☆
BEST TAKEN AS Infusion ✓✓✓ Tincture ✓✓
Tablet ✓
DOSAGE C (*see pp.44–45*)
CAUTIONS Do not take during pregnancy. See also pp.42–51.

Anxiety, nervous exhaustion, and headache Betony tincture or infusion has particular application in chronic nervous states involving mental overactivity. It will help to relieve anxiety and irritability, as well as accompanying symptoms such as poor concentration and headache. It may also be taken for dizziness and nerve pain.

FLOWERS

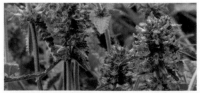

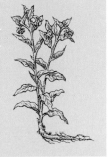

Comfrey

Symphytum officinale

Comfrey root is highly effective in stimulating tissue repair. When applied regularly to damaged tissue such as sprains, bruises, sports injuries, and operation scars, it promotes regrowth and shortens recovery or repair time. Comfrey ointment or cream merits a place in every home first aid kit.

MEDICINAL USES

Parts used Leaf ● Root

Key actions Anti-inflammatory ● Astringent ● Demulcent ● Wound healer

Bruises, sprains, and tissue repair

Applied as soon as possible to the site of bruises, sprains, or minor fractures, comfrey cream or ointment will often minimize swelling and promote quick and effective repair. Continue applying, as ointment, cream, or poultice of leaves and root, until tissue is healed. Comfrey also helps with varicose veins, slow-healing wounds, and ulcers. Where the wound is still open, apply comfrey carefully around the margins of the wound, not directly on it. Apply comfrey with caution during pregnancy.

KEY INFORMATION

SAFETY	★ ★ ★ ★ ☆
TRADITIONAL USE	★ ★ ★ ★ ★
RESEARCH	★ ★ ★ ☆ ☆

BEST TAKEN AS Ointment ✓✓✓
Leaves, cream, lotion ✓✓
DOSAGE T, Leaf: C (*see pp.44–45*)
OFTEN USED WITH Yarrow (*Achillea millefolium*)
CAUTIONS Do not take comfrey root internally. Do not take comfrey leaf internally during pregnancy, or for more than 6 weeks at a time. Do not apply comfrey to open wounds. Restricted in some countries, such as US; internal use not legal in Australia. See also pp.41–52.

root helps to heal bruises   **FRESH ROOT**

Comfrey, which is also known as "knitbone," stimulates bone repair.

Chickweed

Stellaria media

Best known as a remedy for itchy skin, chickweed can also bring relief to problems such as eczema, nettle rash, and irritated varicose veins.

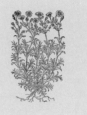

MEDICINAL USES

Part used Whole plant

Key actions Astringent ● Cooling (topically) ● Demulcent ● Relieves itchiness

KEY INFORMATION

SAFETY	★ ★ ★ ⯪ ☆
TRADITIONAL USE	★ ★ ★ ★ ☆
RESEARCH	★ ☆ ☆ ☆ ☆
DOSAGE	T (see pp.44–45)
BEST TAKEN AS	Cream ✓✓✓
Freshly squeezed juice ✓✓	

CAUTIONS Can cause allergic skin reactions; try a small quantity first. See also pp.42–51.

Itchy skin The cream and freshly squeezed juice are markedly cooling on the skin and can be applied as often as needed to soothe sore and itchy areas. The infusion can be added to a bath or cooled and used as a wash on varicose veins.

CREEPING PLANT

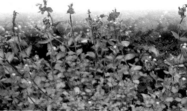

Stevia

Stevia rebaudiana

Stevia is a non-sugar natural sweetener that lowers blood sugar levels and makes a good replacement for both sugar and artificial sweeteners.

MEDICINAL USES

Part used Leaf

Key actions Antimicrobial ● Hypoglycemic (lowers blood sugar levels) ● Lowers blood pressure

Sugar replacement The herb's sweet taste and hypoglycemic action make it a valuable remedy in early onset diabetes. It can also help to prevent tooth decay, aid weight loss, and improve immune resistance in yeast infections. Take on its own as a tea or use in place of sugar—¼ teaspoon of ground leaf is roughly equivalent to 1 teaspoon of sugar.

leaves are sweet-tasting

FRESH LEAVES

KEY INFORMATION

SAFETY	★ ★ ★ ★ ⯪
TRADITIONAL USE	★ ★ ★ ★ ☆
RESEARCH	★ ★ ★ ★ ☆
BEST TAKEN AS	Infusion ✓✓✓
DOSAGE	Food, C (see pp.44–45)

CAUTIONS Avoid during pregnancy. May occasionally cause gastrointestinal upset, headache, or dizziness. See also pp.42–51.

Feverfew

Tanacetum parthenium

A cooling, bitter remedy that was once used to treat fever, feverfew is now a standard remedy for tension headache and migraine. Research, which has by and large confirmed the herb's effectiveness, began after a Welsh doctor's wife found feverfew cured her 50-year-long history of migraine.

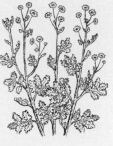

MEDICINAL USES

Part used Leaf

Key actions Anti-inflammatory ● Bitter

Headache and migraine Feverfew proves most effective when it is taken as soon as signs of an impending migraine attack are recognized. The herb is generally less effective once the migraine is underway. The leaf can be used symptomatically, for example, in tension headache. But for best results, the herb should be taken regularly for several months. Strong-acting and potentially toxic, feverfew should be taken at the recommended dosage—either one small fresh leaf with food or as a capsule or tablet produced to pharmacopoeial standards.

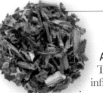

dried leaves are taken to relieve migraine

DRIED LEAVES

Arthritic pain The herb's anti-inflammatory action is useful in treating arthritic aches and pain. It is most likely to relieve arthritic pain when combined with herbs such as willow bark (*Salix alba*) or devil's claw (*Harpogophytum procumbens*).

KEY INFORMATION

SAFETY	★ ★ ★ ⯪ ☆
TRADITIONAL USE	★ ★ ★ ★ ☆
RESEARCH	★ ★ ★ ⯪ ☆

BEST TAKEN AS Tablet ✓✓✓ Capsule ✓✓ Fresh leaf ✓

DOSAGE Tablet, capsule: M *(see pp.44–45)*; one small fresh leaf a day.

CAUTIONS Avoid during pregnancy or while breast-feeding. If taking blood-thinning medication, take only on the advice of a herbal or medical practitioner. Can cause allergic reactions, mouth ulcers, and gastrointestinal upset. See also pp.42–51.

Other uses Feverfew has many traditional uses and has often been

DECOCTION

used to treat hot and feverish states. A strong bitter, it stimulates appetite and digestive activity and has been employed to treat worms. The leaf acts to stimulate menstrual blood flow and can prove helpful in relieving menstrual pains.

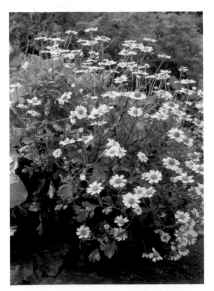

Feverfew has white and yellow daisy-type flowers, and care must be taken not to confuse chamomile (*Chamomilla recutita*) with this potentially toxic herb.

Pau d'arco, Lapacho

Tabebuia spp.

A traditional South American remedy, pau d'arco is thought to be specific for problems such as yeast infection and candidiasis—applied to the skin or taken internally.

MEDICINAL USES

Part used Bark

Key actions Antibacterial ● Antifungal ● Astringent ● Immune-stimulant ● Reputed antitumor activity

Fungal and bacterial infection Best taken in combination with other herbs such as echinacea (*Echinacea* spp.) or goldenseal (*Hydrastis canadensis*)

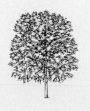

PAU D'ARCO TREE

to treat digestive infections, tonsillitis, thrush and candidiasis, it is used in Brazil as a preventative and adjuvant in cancer treatment (unsupported by research).

KEY INFORMATION

SAFETY   ★ ★ ★ ✭ ☆
TRADITIONAL USE   ★ ★ ★ ★ ★
RESEARCH   ★ ★ ★ ☆ ☆
BEST TAKEN AS Decoction ✓✓✓
Tincture ✓✓ Capsule ✓
DOSAGE C (*see pp.44–45*)
CAUTIONS Do not take during pregnancy. If on prescribed anticoagulant medication, take only on the advice of an herbal or medical practitioner. See also pp.42–51.

Tamarind

Tamarindus indica

Best known for its tart, slightly spicy flavor in chutneys and sauces, tamarind is mainly used as a gentle laxative to treat constipation in children.

MEDICINAL USES

Part used Fruit

Key actions Laxative ● Nutritive

Constipation Fresh or dried fruit can be made into a pleasant drink and

taken to help open the bowels and relieve constipation.

Other uses Recent research has found that the fruit increases the availability of ibuprofen in the body, suggesting that it could be used in arthritis to reduce the dosage of aspirin-type medicines.

TAMARIND TREE

KEY INFORMATION

SAFETY   ★ ★ ★ ★ ✭
TRADITIONAL USE   ★ ★ ✭ ☆ ☆
RESEARCH   ★ ★ ☆ ☆ ☆
BEST TAKEN AS Fruit ✓✓✓
DOSAGE Food, M (*see pp.44–45*)
CAUTIONS May interact with aspirin-type medicines. See also pp.42–51.

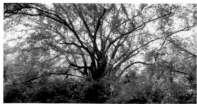

Dandelion

Taraxacum officinalis

One of nature's most versatile remedies, dandelion is both a nutritious salad vegetable and a detoxifying remedy for the liver and kidneys. Loved by herbalists for its gentle cleansing effect, dandelion root finds use in toxic states of all kinds, including chronic skin disorders and recurrent infection.

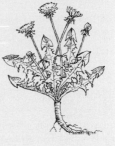

MEDICINAL USES

Parts used Root ● Leaf

Key actions Bitter tonic ● Diuretic ● Liver cleanser ● Mild laxative

Poor appetite and digestion, poor liver function Bitter but not excessively so, dandelion root has a beneficial action on the stomach, liver, and pancreas, increasing digestive secretions, including bile, and tending to stabilize blood sugar levels. The root promotes liver detoxification.

Fluid retention, high blood pressure The standard herbal diuretic, dandelion leaf acts mainly on the kidneys and encourages fluid clearance and weight loss. It is commonly taken to help lower blood pressure, its high potassium content making it particularly useful.

Skin problems A gentle "blood cleanser," dandelion root will prove helpful in a number of chronic skin complaints such as acne, boils, and eczema, especially when it is combined with herbs such as burdock (*Arctium lappa*) and echinacea (*Echinacea* spp.). The leaves are cleansing and nutritious, and make a good addition to salads.

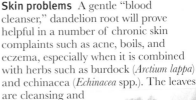

A good diuretic, dandelion is also known as piss-a-bed.

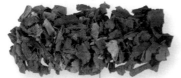

DRIED ROOT | root gently stimulates appetite

KEY INFORMATION

SAFETY ★ ★ ★ ★ ★
TRADITIONAL USE ★ ★ ★ ★ ☆
RESEARCH ★ ★ ★ ☆ ☆
BEST TAKEN AS Root: Tincture ✓✓✓
Leaf: Infusion ✓✓✓ Tincture ✓✓
DOSAGE A (*see pp.44–45*)
OFTEN USED WITH Burdock (*Arctium lappa*)
CAUTIONS Occasionally can cause allergic reaction. See also pp.42–51.

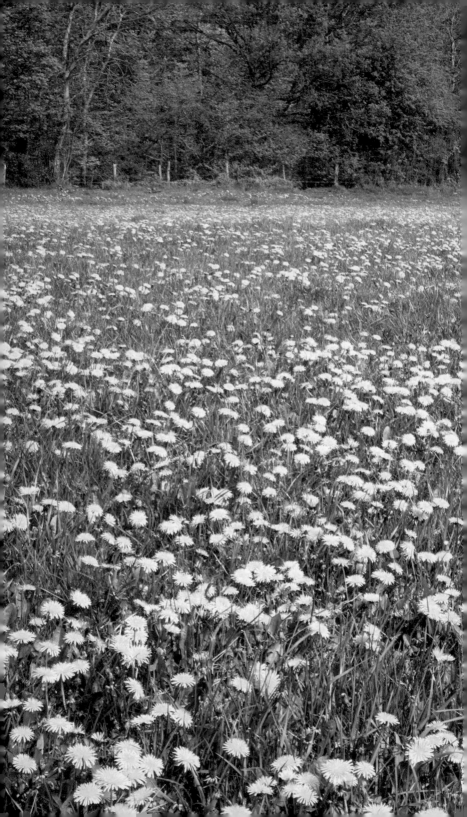

Growing wild in most parts of the world, dandelion (*Taraxacum officinalis*) leaf makes a nutritious addition to salads. Rich in vitamins A and C and iron, the leaf supports liver and kidney function.

Cacoa, Chocolate

Theobroma cacao

For the Mayas, cacoa or chocolate was "the food of the gods." More a food than a medicine, it offers distinct health benefits. Traditionally used as a heart and kidney tonic, dark chocolate is today recommended as an antioxidant for cardiovascular health.

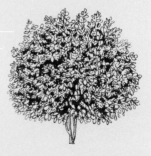

MEDICINAL USES

Part used Seed

Key actions Antioxidant ● Diuretic ● Mild bitter ● Nutritive ● Stimulant

Mood enhancement Due in part to an influence on serotonin and endorphin levels, cacoa induces subtle effects on the mind and emotions, increasing alertness while calming and relaxing the body. Moderate amounts of plain chocolate will enhance mood and support a positive mental state. Overall, cacoa induces a sense of well-being and, as part of a broad approach, can help to lift lowered mood, especially when linked to nervous exhaustion. Where it is difficult to maintain a moderate intake, for example, in premenstrual sugar-craving, other remedies such as damiana (*Turnera diffusa*) or St. John's wort (*Hypericum perforatum*) may be more appropriate.

Other uses A good addition to the diet to maintain cardiovascular health, cocoa or dark chocolate at the end

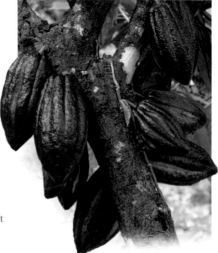

Applied locally, the "butter" extracted from cacoa beans helps to nourish and protect the skin and mucus membranes.

of a meal stimulates digestive activity. Its polyphenols exert an antioxidant activity within the heart and stomach. Research has shown that cacoa helps counter bacteria that cause septicaemia and boils. Cacoa butter is also widely used in making cosmetic preparations, lip salves, and pessaries.

beans contain a nutritious oil

BEANS IN A POD

KEY INFORMATION

SAFETY	★ ★ ★ ★ ★
TRADITIONAL USE	★ ★ ★ ★ ☆
RESEARCH	★ ★ ★ ★ ☆
BEST TAKEN AS	Infusion ✓✓✓
Plain chocolate ✓✓	
DOSAGE	Food

CAUTIONS Can cause migraine headache and gastrointestinal upset. See also pp.42–51.

roasted beans are used to make chocolate

ROASTED BEANS

Thuja, Tree of life

Thuja occidentalis

Native Americans employed thuja for conditions such as headache, fever, and rheumatism, and burned it as a cleansing "smudge." Thuja's main application is for warts, though it helps in other infectious conditions as well—notably sinusitis, tooth abscesses, bronchitis, cystitis, and fungal infections.

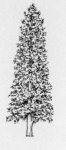

MEDICINAL USES

Part used Leaf

Key actions Antifungal ● Antimicrobial ● Antiviral ● Blood cleanser

Warts and topical application No remedy is guaranteed to remove warts, but thuja is more likely to succeed than many others. Apply neat tincture to the wart twice a day. Continue for up to 10 days.

Infections Not normally taken on its own, thuja combines well with other antimicrobial and immune-enhancing remedies, notably echinacea (*Echinacea* spp.) and thyme (*Thymus vulgaris*). Its marked antiseptic activity is most apparent in viral and bacterial infections affecting mucous membranes, especially membranes within the ear, nose, throat, and urinary tract. Strong-acting and potentially toxic when taken internally, thuja is best used on professional advice.

LEAVES

Other uses Thuja is prescribed by practitioners for a wide variety of conditions, including psoriasis, fibroids, and bedwetting. It has been prescribed for uterine polyps and uterine cancer, which can be caused by the wart virus that produces polyps. In rheumatic problems, a lotion can be applied topically as a counterirritant to relieve muscular aches and pains.

Thuja contains a strong volatile oil with potent antifungal and antiviral acitivity.

leaves can be used to treat warts

KEY INFORMATION

SAFETY	★★★☆☆
TRADITIONAL USE	★★★★☆
RESEARCH	★★★☆☆
BEST TAKEN AS	Tincture ✓✓✓
DOSAGE	D (see pp.44–45)
OFTEN USED WITH	Echinacea (*Echinacea* spp.)

CAUTIONS Do not take thuja during pregnancy and while breast-feeding. See also pp.42–51.

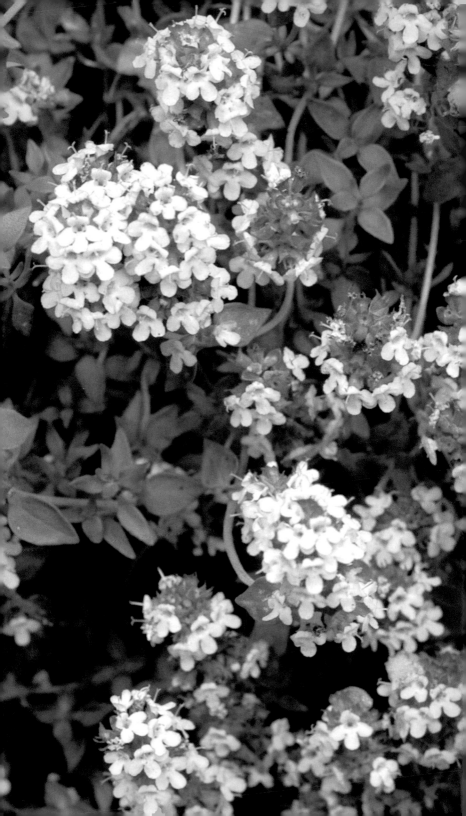

A much-loved kitchen herb with medicinal activity, thyme (*Thymus vulgaris*) flowers are a favorite of bees. Honey produced from the flowers is prized for its rich and distinctive flavor.

Thyme, Common thyme

Thymus vulgaris

A classic kitchen herb, thyme makes a refreshing tea that counters infection and tones the respiratory system. Useful in almost any problem affecting the ear, nose, throat, and chest, thyme disinfects the air passages, soothes coughing, and stimulates clearance of phlegm.

MEDICINAL USES

Parts used Aerial parts

Key actions Antibacterial ● Antifungal ● Antioxidant ● Expectorant ● Relaxant ● Tonic

FRESH LEAVES

Ear, nose, and throat (ENT) problems Thyme tea, with or without a spoonful of honey, is an excellent home remedy for ENT problems, including colds, catarrh, sinus congestion, sore throat, and tonsillitis. The tea can be used first as a gargle and then swallowed.

Cough and bronchial infection Thyme brings relief to all manners of cough and chest problems, and can provide valuable support in asthma and whooping cough. It is often combined with licorice (*Glycyrrhiza glabra*) and echinacea (*Echinacea* spp.).

Other uses The tea may be taken as a general tonic, as well as to relieve indigestion and gas and to treat threadworms. In arthritic and rheumatic conditions, it makes an invigorating addition to a bath. The essential oil can be applied undiluted to fungally-infected nails; use 1 drop per nail twice a day (do not use undiluted elsewhere and do not take internally).

KEY INFORMATION

SAFETY	★ ★ ★ ★ ☆
TRADITIONAL USE	★ ★ ★ ★ ☆
RESEARCH	★ ★ ★ ☆ ☆

BEST TAKEN AS Infusion ✓✓✓ Tincture ✓✓
DOSAGE C (*see pp.44–45*)
OFTEN USED WITH Licorice (*Glycyrrhiza glabra*)
CAUTIONS Rarely, may cause gastrointestinal upset or allergic reaction. See also pp.42–51.

DRIED AERIAL PARTS

Traditionally, thyme is seen as a "longevity" herb, a view supported by evidence that it prevents the breakdown of essential fatty acids within the brain.

Puncture vine, Caltrops

Tribulus terrestris

This plant has been used for at least 2,000 years in both western and eastern traditions as a remedy for kidney and bladder problems, particularly kidney stones. It also possesses a longstanding reputation as a tonic and aphrodisiac.

MEDICINAL USES

Parts used Flower ● Fruit ● Root

Key actions Anti-inflammatory ● Estrogenic ● Reputed aphrodisiac ● Stimulates menstruation

Kidney and urinary tract problems
A useful remedy for urinary problems such as cystitis and urethritis, puncture vine can be particularly helpful for the chronic urethral irritation that quite often occurs as estrogen levels fall at the time of menopause. In combination with other remedies, it has been commonly used to help clear kidney and bladder stones, though for these conditions it needs to be taken after professional advice.

Sexual tonic A tonic for both men and women, puncture vine is likely to help most where sexual vitality and libido are at a low ebb. In women it can help to improve libido, especially during menopause, and in men there are indications that it can help with problems such as erectile dysfunction and lowered testosterone levels.

Body building Currently in vogue as a body-building supplement, puncture vine

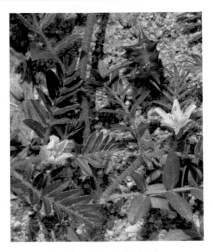

Puncture vine thrives on waste land. A thorny, creeping plant, it can be found growing all the way from south-eastern Europe to China.

contains steroidal saponins, which are thought to increase muscle bulk in much the same way as testosterone. Despite the hype surrounding the herb, the root and leaf clearly do have hormonal activity within the body, though are probably only effective (anabolic) when testosterone levels are low.

KEY INFORMATION

SAFETY   ★ ★ ★ ⯪ ☆
TRADITIONAL USE   ★ ★ ★ ★ ☆
RESEARCH   ★ ★ ☆ ☆ ☆
BEST TAKEN AS Tablet ✓✓✓
Capsule ✓✓
DOSAGE M (*see pp.44–45*)
CAUTIONS Keep to recommended dosage.
Avoid during pregnancy. See also pp.42–51.

fruit contains steroidal saponins

CAPSULES   **FRUIT**

Limeflower, Linden blossom

Tilia spp.

Commonly planted in gardens and parks, the lime or linden tree bears flowers that perfume the air on summer evenings. The delicate scent acts much in the same way as the infusion made from the flowers, soothing troubled states of mind and relieving tension headaches, migraines, and sinus congestion.

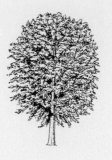

MEDICINAL USES

Part used Flower

Key actions Antispasmodic
● Diaphoretic ● Mild sedative
● Nerve tonic

Colds, catarrh, and fever Limeflower is considered to be an excellent remedy for head colds and mild fevers, as well as nasal or sinus catarrh; drink small amounts of limeflower tea frequently throughout the day. It is an excellent remedy for children, and can be blended with some apple juice in order to improve the taste. The tea also makes a good steam inhalation to ease sinus headache and congestion. Limeflower combines well with elderflower (*Sambucus nigra*).

Native to Europe, the lime tree is found in the wild. These trees grow up to 100ft (30m), with heart-shaped leaves and clusters of yellow flowers.

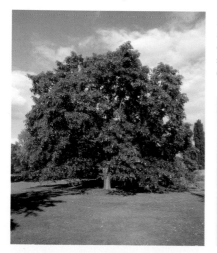

Anxiety and tension Under-appreciated, perhaps because it is a gentle-acting remedy, limeflower has constituents that exert a mild tranquilizing effect, similar in some respects to benzodiazepine tranquilizers (for example, Xanax or Valium). Usually best taken as an infusion or tincture, limeflower helps to cool and relieve anxiety states, particularly when symptoms include head and neck tension, palpitations, and feeling "hot and bothered." Its mild action makes it valuable in helping to soothe agitation and restlessness in children, and it can also be taken to calm emotional shock, combining well here with oat straw (*Avena sativa*).

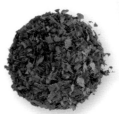

DRIED FLOWERS

Poor sleep A good nighttime drink, limeflower tea is safe for children and adults alike, encouraging relaxation and a drift into sleep rather than being overly sedative. Combine with passion flower (*Passiflora incarnata*) to increase the sedative

KEY INFORMATION

SAFETY	★ ★ ★ ★ ✬
TRADITIONAL USE	★ ★ ★ ★ ☆
RESEARCH	★ ★ ★ ☆ ☆
BEST TAKEN AS	Infusion ✓ ✓ ✓
DOSAGE	B (*see pp.44–45*)
OFTEN USED WITH	Hawthorn

(*Crataegus* spp.)

CAUTIONS Can occasionally cause allergic reactions. Pollen can provoke hay fever. See also pp.42–51.

The father of modern botany and ecology, Carl Linné or Linnaeus (1707–1778) reputedly owed his name to the lime tree that grew by his family home.

strength of the tea. For nervous tension and to aid sleep, 50–300g (2–10oz) of flowers can be infused for 20 minutes in the evening and added to a warm bath. Relax and soak in the bath, then retire to bed.

Palpitations and high blood pressure

Specifically used for nervous palpitations, the flowers are thought to slow and stabilize the heart rate and rhythm and are often prescribed by herbal practitioners for an irregular or racing heartbeat. Limeflower can also be valuable as part of a broad approach to treating high blood pressure, especially where this is associated with arteriosclerosis (hardening of the arteries) and nervous tension. Taken long-term, limeflower's high bio-flavonoid content helps to improve the health of the arteries, and the flowers combine particularly well with hawthorn (*Crataegus* spp.) to support healthy heart function and circulation.

Other uses Limeflower stimulates blood flow to the capillaries and surface of the body, thereby stimulating sweating and

LIMEFLOWER HONEY

"Bees are extremely fond of flowers of the lime, which abound with honey, and they also sometimes collect the sweet 'honey dew', the deposit of aphids, that covers the leaves during summer. In Lithuania, holes are made in large trees, which the bees soon convert into hives and the combs are removed when full. Such honey is thought a valuable remedy in Poland for lung disorders, and fetches a very high price."
C. Pierpoint
Johnson,
1875

HONEY BEE

helping to cool the body in hot and feverish states. When combined with circulatory stimulants such as ginkgo (*Ginkgo biloba*) or angelica (*Angelica archangelica*), this circulatory effect can help to improve peripheral circulation and a tendency to cold extremities. Conditions such as chilblains and restless legs can also benefit.

Red clover

Trifolium pratense

Traditionally seen as a "hot" and "dry" herb, red clover's dense red flowers were thought in medieval times to signify its value as a blood cleanser. Taken to clear chronic toxicity, red clover is an important remedy for skin problems such as acne, boils, eczema, and psoriasis.

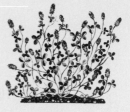

MEDICINAL USES

Part used Flower

Key actions Antispasmodic
- Blood cleanser • Expectorant
- Phytoestrogenic
- Reputed anticancer activity

Chronic toxicity A mild laxative, red clover is most likely to aid detoxification in cases where skin and glandular problems are linked with chronic constipation. Safe for children with mild skin conditions or swollen glands linked to a sore throat, red clover works best with small doses initially that are slowly increased. It combines well with other skin remedies, including echinacea (*Echinacea* spp.). The herb's use as an anticancer remedy is unsubstantiated, though its ability to stimulate cleansing of the lymph system suggests that it may have a role as an adjuvant along with herbs such as yellow dock (*Rumex crispus*). Red clover also works well with herbs such as marigold (*Calendula officinalis*) to ease swollen and painful breasts, but concentrated extracts

INFUSION | infusion supports skin health

should not be taken during pregnancy and while breast-feeding.

Chest problems Traditionally given to children as a remedy for chest coughs and wheeziness, red clover can prove useful in chest problems, especially when combined with thyme (*Thymus vulgaris*). Taken as a hot tea sweetened with honey, this combination can help to soothe chronic and irritable coughs and may be helpful alongside prescribed medication for problems such as bronchitis and bronchial asthma. Red clover has also been used to treat night sweats associated with chest infection.

KEY INFORMATION

SAFETY	★ ★ ★ ★ ✬
TRADITIONAL USE	★ ★ ★ ★ ☆
RESEARCH	★ ★ ☆ ☆ ☆

BEST TAKEN AS Tincture ✓✓✓
Infusion ✓✓ Capsule, tablet ✓
DOSAGE A *(see pages 44–45)*
OFTEN USED WITH Yellow dock
(*Rumex crispus*)
CAUTIONS Rarely, can cause headache or skin rash. Do not take concentrated extracts during pregnancy and while breast-feeding. See also pp.41–52.

flowers promote detoxification

DRIED FLOWERS

THE CLOVER LEAF

Many classical stories and myths relate to the clover. Perhaps the most enduring legacy of these myths concerns the "club" of our playing cards, said to resemble a clover leaf. The clover leaf in turn resembles the three-lobed club wielded by Hercules, known in Latin as *clava trinodis*.

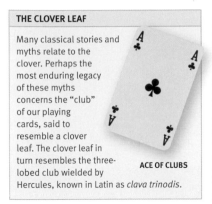

ACE OF CLUBS

circulation. However, concentrated extracts such as these are very different from typical herbal preparations, and need to be seen as separate products with distinct areas of activity. In view of the high levels of phyoestrogens present, it is advisable to take concentrated isoflavone extracts up to a maximum of 3 months at a time. Where repeated use is desired, it is best to seek professional advice.

FRESH HERB

Menopausal symptoms Concentrated isoflavone extracts that are strongly estrogenic are available over-the-counter as an alternative form of hormone replacement therapy. They can prove helpful in relieving menopausal symptoms that are usually linked to lowered estrogen levels, such as hot flashes, night sweats, headaches, and poor sleep. Due to the high levels of isoflavone, concentrated extracts also have anti-inflammatory activity and support the health of the heart and

Other uses A lotion made from the tea makes a useful skin wash for persistent sores, inflamed skin, and swollen insect bites. The flowers may also be decocted, strained, and while warm applied as a poultice on swollen and tender glands.

In Spain, red clover was traditionally used to help in treating cataracts. The pale crescent marking on the herb's leaves was thought to resemble a cataract.

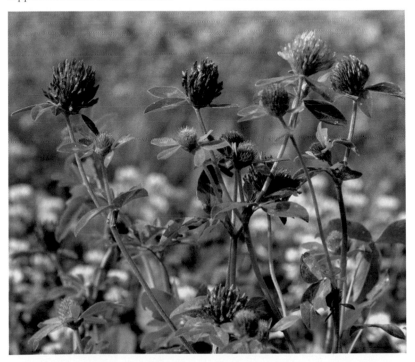

A common wayside and meadow plant, red clover (*Trifolium pratense*) has pink, oval-shaped flower heads, which in the past were gathered and used for dyeing wool green.

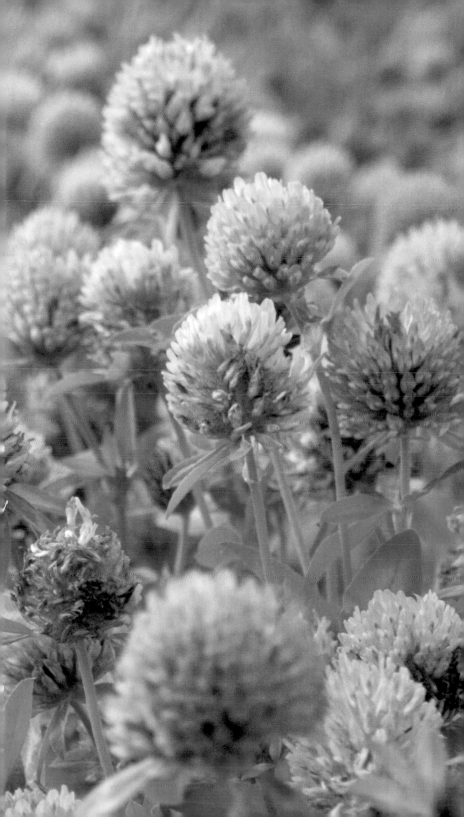

Fenugreek

Trigonella foenum-graecum

Strongly mucilaginous, fenugreek soothes and heals sore, inflamed, or ulcerated tissue in the gastrointestinal tract. Clinical trials have shown that it lowers levels of "bad" fats, like cholesterol, LDL, VLDL, and triglycerides, within the blood. Blood sugar control and insulin response in diabetics are also improved.

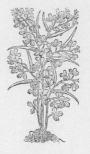

MEDICINAL USES

Parts used   Seed ● Sprout

Key actions   Anti-inflammatory ● Demulcent ● Expectorant ● Laxative ● Lowers cholesterol and blood sugar levels

Gastrointestinal problems   Inflammatory problems within the digestive tract such as mouth ulcers, gastritis, and irritable bowel will benefit from the seeds' moistening and protective effect. For best results, first soak the seeds in water.

Cholesterol and blood sugar

Clinical evidence supports fenugreek's use in raised cholesterol levels; however, large doses were used in the clinical trials (5–100g a day)

to achieve this result. The seeds can also be used on a daily basis to help reduce blood sugar levels in diabetes. Components in fenugreek stimulate insulin as well as delay absorption of glucose.

Fenugreek seeds are strongly estrogenic and can be valuable in menopausal symptoms.

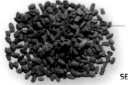

seeds have a demulcent action

SEEDS

KEY INFORMATION

SAFETY	★★★★⯨
TRADITIONAL USE	★★★★☆
RESEARCH	★★★⯨☆

BEST TAKEN AS Ground or sprouting seeds ✓✓✓ Decoction ✓✓ Capsule ✓

DOSAGE A (*see pp.44–45*)

CAUTIONS During pregnancy, or if taking prescribed anticoagulant or diabetic medication, take only on the advice of an herbal or medical practitioner. Occasionally can cause gastrointestinal upset. See also pp.42–51.

Damiana

Turnera diffusa, T. aphrodisiaca

Renowned as a tonic that enhances vitality and lifts mood, damiana is thought to have aphrodisiac qualities that stimulate libido in men and women.

MEDICINAL USES

Part used Leaf

Key actions Mild antidepressant
- Nerve tonic ● Reputed aphrodisiac
- Urinary antiseptic

KEY INFORMATION

SAFETY　　　　　　★ ★ ★ ★ ☆
TRADITIONAL USE　★ ★ ★ ★ ☆
RESEARCH　　　　 ★ ★ ☆ ☆ ☆
BEST TAKEN AS Infusion ✓✓✓ Iincture ✓✓ Capsule ✓
DOSAGE B (*see pp.44–45*)
CAUTIONS None known. See also pp.42–51

Nervous exhaustion, mild depression
Taken regularly, damiana will help to improve mood and mental stamina. It is best taken in combination with herbs such as skullcap (*Scutellaria lateriflora*) or St. John's wort (*Hypericum perforatum*).

Sexual tonic A gentle acting remedy, damiana is a useful restorative. It can be safely taken to enhance the libido in both men and women.

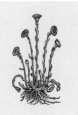

FLOWER

Coltsfoot

Tussilago farafara

An excellent remedy for irritable coughs and catarrh, coltsfoot soothes and relaxes the chest, eases breathing, and aids the coughing up of mucus.

MEDICINAL USES

Part used Leaf

Key actions Anticatarrhal
● Demulcent ● Expectorant

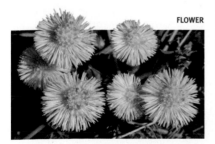

FLOWER

Cough and chest problems Coltsfoot acts to counter inflammation and clear congestion. It can be put to good use in painful cough, wheeziness, chronic bronchitis, and emphysema.

KEY INFORMATION

SAFETY　　　　　　★ ★ ★ ★ ☆
TRADITIONAL USE　★ ★ ★ ⯨ ☆
RESEARCH　　　　 ★ ★ ☆ ☆ ☆
BEST TAKEN AS Standardized extract ✓✓✓
DOSAGE M (*see pp.44–45*)
CAUTIONS Do not take during pregnancy and while breast-feeding. Take only standardized products. Restricted herb in some countries, including Australia. See also pp.42–51.

Slippery elm

Ulmus fulva

Few herbs are more valued in Western herbal medicine than slippery elm. Readily digestible, the powdered bark can be mixed with water to form a thick jelly-like solution that has limitless applications, whether topically on the skin or internally within the gastrointestinal tract.

MEDICINAL USES

Part used   Root (powdered) ● Bark

Key actions   Antioxidant ● Demulcent ● Emollient ● Nutritive

Digestive and respiratory problems

Slippery elm soothes and protects in problems such as heartburn, irritable bowel, and bronchitis. Stir 1–2 teaspoonfuls of powder into water and leave to stand for 5 minutes before drinking. Add a pinch of cinnamon powder, if wanted. Repeat as desired. Be sure to buy slippery elm powder, and not wheat powder with added slippery elm. Avoid taking slippery elm with other medications as it tends to reduce absorption.

Topical uses   As a "drawing" poultice for splinters, boils, and ulcers, mix a small quantity of slippery elm with echinacea (*Echinacea* spp.) infusion or tincture to form a thick paste. Spread onto the affected area and bandage. Leave for 24 hours. Repeat as required.

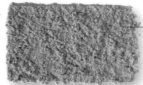

powdered root soothes inflammation

POWDERED ROOT

KEY INFORMATION

SAFETY   ★ ★ ★ ★ ★
TRADITIONAL USE   ★ ★ ★ ★ ★
RESEARCH   ★ ★ ★ ☆ ☆
BEST TAKEN AS Powdered root (mixed with water) ✓✓✓
DOSAGE A (*see pp.44–45*)
OFTEN USED WITH Echinacea (*Echinacea purpurea*)
CAUTIONS Use only inner bark. Mix powder with plenty of water. Rarely, may cause local irritation. See also pp.42–51.

Slippery elm coats the inner lining of the stomach and intestines, relieving acidity, irritability, and inflammation.

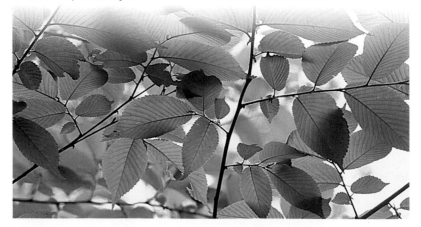

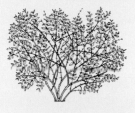

Cat's claw, Una de gato

Uncaria tomentosa

A climbing vine native to the Amazon rainforest, cat's claw is believed by local healers to have great medicinal virtue; they use it as a cure-all to treat everything from asthma and arthritis to diabetes and cancer. It is an endangered species in the wild; use organic products only.

MEDICINAL USES

Part used Stem bark ● Root

Key actions Anti-inflammatory ● Antioxidant ● Immune tonic

Chronic infection Cat's claw's tonic action on the immune system makes it a key remedy for chronic infection and degenerative diseases. Best taken combined with other immune-enhancing herbs, cat's claw can

DRIED BARK

KEY INFORMATION

SAFETY	★ ★ ★ ✬ ☆
TRADITIONAL USE	★ ★ ★ ★ ★
RESEARCH	★ ★ ★ ☆ ☆

BEST TAKEN AS Tincture ✓✓✓ Tablets (preferably organic standardized) ✓✓
DOSAGE B (*see pp.44–45*)
OFTEN USED WITH Echinacea (*Echinacea purpurea*)
CAUTIONS Do not take during pregnancy and while breast-feeding. May have contraceptive activity. Take on the advice of a herbal or medical practitioner if on blood-thinning or immunosuppressant medication. Can cause nausea or headache. See also pp.42–51.

Cat's claw helps to boost the immune system, and is also useful in gastrointestinal infection and inflammation.

inflammatory joint problems such as osteo- and rheumatoid arthritis.

Anticancer remedy Reflecting its traditional South American use, cat's claw has antitumor properties that make it valuable as an adjuvant treatment in cancer. Take with other appropriate herbal medicines and on professional advice.

THE "CAT'S CLAW"

prove useful in treating chronic fatigue, fibromyalgia, mononucleosis, and herpes infection. Clinical studies in Peru suggest the herb can be helpful in HIV infection. It is a first-rate convalescent herb.

Anti-inflammatory Cat's claw has potent anti-inflammatory activity and can be successfully used to treat problems such as gastric ulceration, as well as

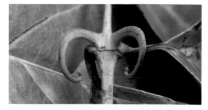

Nettle

Urtica dioica, U. urens

Infamous for its stinging leaves, nettle is a fine example of a weed that has great value as food and medicine. Rich in iron, calcium, and silica, nettle leaf makes a useful tonic food—as tea or soup—in anemia and rheumatic problems. Nettle leaf also has marked anti-allergenic activity.

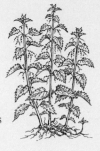

MEDICINAL USES

Parts used Aerial parts ● Root

Key actions Anti-allergenic ● Anti-inflammatory ● Antispasmodic (root) ● Blood cleanser ● Diuretic ● Tonic (leaf)

Arthritic and rheumatic problems

Nettle's primary use is for stiff and inflamed joints, with conditions such as gout benefiting especially. Taken long-term for arthritic and rheumatic symptoms, nettle leaf can relieve pain and inflammation and support tissue repair. A safe remedy, nettle leaf tea or soup can be taken in relatively large amounts to maximize its anti-inflammatory activity. In a German clinical trial, patients with osteoarthritis were able to significantly reduce their intake of aspirin-type anti-inflammatories on taking nettle leaf. High levels of histamine and serotonin in the stinging hairs are thought to be

juice of leaves
cures nettle sting

root has
diuretic effect

FRESH AERIAL PARTS   **FRESH ROOT**

responsible for the herb's "sting," and may explain the ancient practice of flaying an arthritic joint with nettle leaves (*U. urens*) in order to treat pain and stiffness. This traditional use of nettle received unexpected confirmation in a recent double blind clinical trial.

Skin disorders A good detox remedy, nettle leaf combines well with other herbs such as calendula (*Calendula officinalis*) and yellow dock (*Rumex crispus*) to treat all manner of chronic skin problems such as eczema, psoriasis, and urticaria. Apply nettle infusion as a lotion to relieve inflamed and weakened skin, as well as on varicose veins.

DRIED AERIAL PARTS

Enlarged prostate Following several clinical studies, nettle root is now commonly used as first-line treatment in Europe to treat symptoms of enlarged prostate such as poor urine flow, pain or difficulty in passing urine, and urinary

KEY INFORMATION

SAFETY	★★★★☆
TRADITIONAL USE	★★★★☆
RESEARCH	★★★☆☆

BEST TAKEN AS Leaf: Infusion ✓✓✓ Soup ✓✓ Tincture ✓ Root: Tincture ✓✓✓ Tablet ✓✓

DOSAGE Leaf and root: A (*see pp.44–45*)

OFTEN USED WITH Calendula (*Calendula officinalis*)

CAUTIONS Fresh plant will sting! Rarely, can cause allergic skin reactions. Avoid root in pregnancy. See also pp.42–51.

NETTLE AS A VEGETABLE

In spring or early summer, put on a pair of gloves and collect fresh young nettles—shoots, stems, and leaves—from unpolluted, unsprayed areas. Remove thick or old stems. Wash thoroughly, place in a non-aluminium saucepan, cover, and simmer for 5 minutes (no added water is needed). Add butter or margarine and salt and pepper as required. Serve warm, puréed in a blender if required. Alternatively, use as a base for nettle soup.

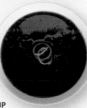

NETTLE SOUP

Found in temperate regions worldwide, nettle has been used medicinally for centuries. The aerial parts are picked in summer, while the shoots are picked in spring and eaten as a tonic food and vegetable.

frequency. Nettle root can be taken on its own as a tincture, or combined with saw palmetto (*Serenoa repens*).

Other uses Taken internally, nettle helps to prevent or stop bleeding from wounds and nosebleeds; it is a valuable remedy for heavy menstrual bleeding, reducing blood loss and, given its appreciable iron content, helping to prevent anemia. Nettle leaf has anti-allergenic activity and is a useful addition to formulations for hay fever and asthma. Nettle leaf infusion makes an effective hair rinse.

NETTLE CAPSULES

Cranberry

Vaccinium macrocarpon

A well-known household remedy, cranberry is commonly taken for urinary tract problems such as cystitis and urethritis. Sharp-flavored and rich in vitamin C, it has strong disinfectant properties within the urinary and gastrointestinal tracts.

MEDICINAL USES

Parts used Fruit ● Juice

Key actions Antioxidant ● Antiseptic

Cystitis and urethritis Cranberry contains constituents which make it difficult for bacteria to cling to the wall of the urinary tubules and intestines so that harmful bacteria are more readily flushed out of the body. Best taken as an unsweetened juice or concentrated extract, cranberry can be combined with other fruit juices, for example apple juice, to make it more palatable. Avoid juices with large amounts of added sugar, not least because sugar depresses the immune system. Clinical research suggests that large quantities can be drunk for acute infection—up to 3 cups a day for a few days, along with plenty of water. For long-term use, take less than half this quantity.

The North American cranberry has been well researched and is now recognized as a safe and effective treatment for mild urinary tract infection.

juice flushes out bacteria

JUICE

Prostate problems Cranberry's tonic and antiseptic action within the urinary tract makes it useful in problems affecting the prostate gland. Taken regularly as a juice or extract, it can help to ease frequency and other symptoms associated with an enlarged prostate. Other prostate problems, such as chronic prostatitis, may benefit from medium to long-term use.

Other uses Cranberry can also be a valuable supplement to take in digestive infections and diarrhea, and in allergic states affecting the gut or respiratory system.

KEY INFORMATION

SAFETY	★ ★ ★ ★ ½
TRADITIONAL USE	★ ★ ★ ½ ☆
RESEARCH	★ ★ ★ ★ ☆

BEST TAKEN AS Unsweetened juice ✓✓✓ Fruit ✓✓ Tablet ✓

DOSAGE A (*see pp.44–45*)

OFTEN USED WITH Buchu (*Barosma betulina*)

CAUTIONS Very high doses may increase effect of prescribed anticoagulant medication, and can cause gastrointestinal upset. See also pp.42–51.

berries are strongly antioxidant

BERRIES

Bilberry, Blueberry

Vaccinium myrtillus

Bilberry tones up small blood vessels, especially capillaries, that permeate the tissues of the body. In particular, bilberry acts on the micro-circulation of the eye and can help to improve night vision and eyesight.

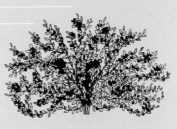

MEDICINAL USES

Parts used Fruit ● Juice ● Leaf

Key actions Anti-inflammatory
● Anti-edema (prevents fluid retention)
● Antioxidant ● Astringent
● Circulatory tonic (fruit) ● Urinary antiseptic (leaf)

Eyesight aid Taken long-term, bilberry improves eye health, protecting against damage to the eye resulting from diabetes and high blood pressure. It can sometimes help in short-sightedness, and in the prevention of cataract formation.

Other uses Bilberry helps to improve poor peripheral circulation and prevents fluid leakage from blood vessels. Many circulatory problems can benefit from taking bilberry, including hemorrhoids and varicose veins, chilblains, Raynaud's disease, intermittent claudication, and easy bruising. Bilberries can be taken to relieve diarrhea or constipation, and the leaves are a useful urinary antiseptic for conditions such as cystitis.

Bilberry's potent antioxidant activity makes it a useful supplement in many chronic health problems, especially where circulation is poor.

KEY INFORMATION

SAFETY	★ ★ ★ ★ ☆
TRADITIONAL USE	★ ★ ★ ★ ☆
RESEARCH	★ ★ ★ ☆ ☆

BEST TAKEN AS Fruit ✓ ✓ ✓ Tincture ✓ ✓ Tablet ✓

DOSAGE A (*see pp. 44–45*)

OFTEN USED WITH Hawthorn (*Crataegus* spp.)

CAUTIONS Very high doses may increase the effect of prescribed anticoagulant medication. See also pp. 42-51.

DRIED LEAVES

berries tone the blood vessels

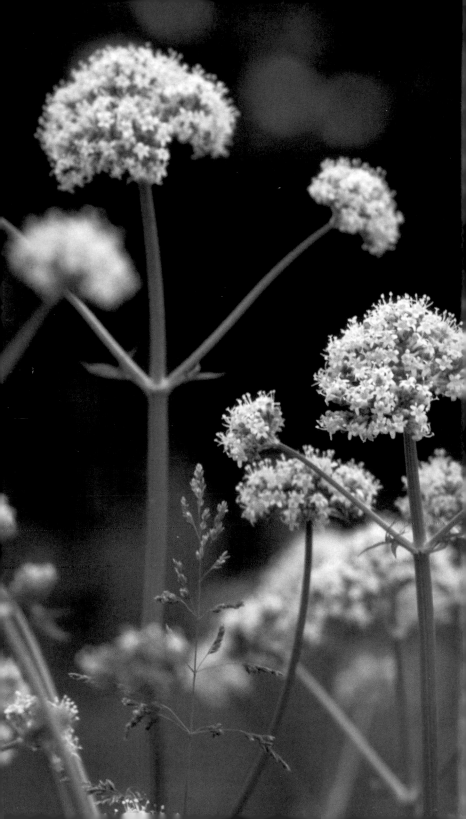

Primarily used as a stress-reliever, valerian (*Valeriana officinalis*) soothes nervous tension and anxiety. Its antispasmodic action works well in muscle pains and digestive cramps.

Valerian

Valeriana officinalis

Used wherever nervous tension, overactivity, or an inability to relax are present, valerian's gently sedative action helps to soothe and slow a nervous system that is beginning to spin out of control. It is one of the first herbs to consider when a remedy is needed to ease anxiety and panic attacks.

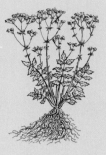

MEDICINAL USES

Part used Root

Key actions Antispasmodic ● Mild analgesic ● Mild bitter ● Tranquillizer

Anxiety, nervous tension Safe and non-addictive, valerian helps in easing anxiety symptoms such as tension headache, palpitations, and tensed muscles. Take valerian on its own or in combination with herbs such as oat straw (*Avena sativa*) or skullcap (*Scutellaria lateriflora*). For nervous palpitations, combine it with limeflower (*Tilia* spp.). People vary in their response to valerian – some feel sedated even with a low dose, but for a few it produces a stimulant effect. Start with a low dose and build up. Valerian is usually best taken in small frequent doses through the day.

KEY INFORMATION

SAFETY	★ ★ ★ ★ ✭
TRADITIONAL USE	★ ★ ★ ★ ✭
RESEARCH	★ ★ ★ ★ ☆

BEST TAKEN AS Tablet ✓✓✓ Capsule ✓✓✓ Tincture ✓✓
DOSAGE B (*see pp.44–45*)
OFTEN USED WITH Skullcap (*Scutellaria lateriflolia*).
CAUTIONS Can cause drowsiness, for example, when driving or using machinery. Rarely, can cause headache or gastrointestinal upset, or worsen anxiety/insomnia. See also pp.42–51.

FRESH ROOT

Poor sleep A key remedy in many herbal sleep preparations, valerian can prove valuable when sleep is disturbed due to worry or overwork. Combined with St. John's wort (*Hypericum perforatum*), it improves sleep quality and eases anxiety and depression.

Other uses A good antispasmodic, valerian can relieve muscle pain and tension in menstrual cramps, rheumatic aches, and irritable bowel syndrome.

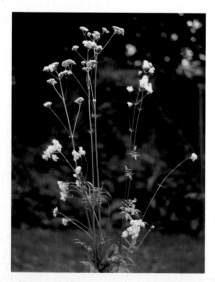

root calms anxiety

DRIED ROOT

Native to Europe and northern Asia, valerian grows in the wild in damp conditions. Its name is thought to be derived from the Latin *valere*, which means "to be well."

Vervain

Verbena officinalis

Used in western and Chinese herbal traditions, vervain is restorative, acting mainly on the nervous and digestive systems. Traditional indications include nervous exhaustion, headaches, migraine, menstrual problems, weak digestive function, and urinary tract infection.

MEDICINAL USES

Parts used Aerial parts

Key actions Mild antidepressant
● Mild digestive tonic ● Nerve tonic
● Relaxant

Anxiety and nervous tension Thought to improve nervous vitality, vervain can be taken where long-term stress and worry are leading to nervous exhaustion. It is a useful remedy for migraine and stress-induced headaches. For best results, it should be taken for several weeks.

Premenstrual problems Thought to have mild progesterogenic activity, vervain is a valuable remedy for premenstrual tension and menstrual headaches, especially when combined with chaste berry (*Vitex agnus-castus*).

Other uses Vervain is an excellent remedy for poor appetite, especially where emotional factors are responsible. Useful therefore in anorexia nervosa, the herb is best taken as a tincture before meals—if necessary, as drops in water or fruit juice. In China, vervain has been used to treat fever, such as in malaria. Although poorly researched, it appears to protect the liver. Vervain tea is taken traditionally to aid breast milk production.

A poorly researched remedy, vervain is prized by herbalists for its ability to restore a depleted nervous system and allay anxiety.

tincture
stimulates
appetite

TINCTURE

KEY INFORMATION

SAFETY	★ ★ ★ ★ ☆
TRADITIONAL USE	★ ★ ★ ★ ☆
RESEARCH	★ ☆ ☆ ☆ ☆

BEST TAKEN AS Infusion ✓✓✓
Tincture ✓✓
DOSAGE B (*see pp.44–45*)
OFTEN USED WITH St. John's wort (*Hypericum perforatum*)
CAUTIONS Rarely, may cause skin rash. See also pp.42–51.

Cramp bark, Guelder rose

Viburnum opulus

Useful in problems affecting both skeletal muscle and internal organs, cramp bark lives up to its reputation as an effective antispasmodic. A key remedy in Western herbal medicine, cramp bark relaxes excessive muscle tone, thereby easing tensed and cramping muscles.

MEDICINAL USES

Part used Bark

Key actions Antispasmodic ● Astringent ● Lowers blood pressure

Muscle cramps and pains Rheumatic pain sometimes results more from locked muscles than inflammation. Here, cramp bark can prove particularly effective, relaxing tensed muscles and opening up the circulation to clear accumulated toxins—often a key factor in pain development. As well as relieving rheumatic and arthritic problems, cramp bark's antispasmodic action makes it a worthwhile treatment for restless legs, leg cramps, and spasmodic period pains. Take on its own to provide symptomatic relief, or combine with anti-inflammatory remedies and circulatory stimulants, such as willow bark (*Salix alba*) and prickly ash (*Zanthoxylum* spp.), for rheumatic problems such as fibromyalgia. For period pains, take the remedy before pain begins.

Digestive cramps Cramp bark is effective for intestinal spasms, including irritable bowel syndrome. It

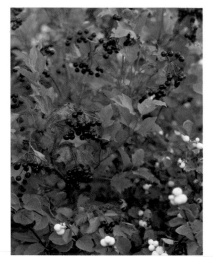

Found growing in hedges, thickets, and woodland, cramp bark has distinctive red berries. It is native to Europe and the eastern regions of North America.

combines well with chamomile (*Chamomilla recutita*) for cramps throughout the gastrointestinal tract.

Other uses Cramp bark is often included in formulations for high blood pressure, especially where tensed muscles are a feature.

tincture is taken to relieve muscle tension

DRIED BARK   **TINCTURE**

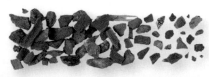

KEY INFORMATION

SAFETY ★★★★★
TRADITIONAL USE ★★★★☆
RESEARCH ★★☆☆☆
BEST TAKEN AS Decoction ✓✓✓ Tincture ✓✓ Capsule ✓
DOSAGE B (*see pp.44–45*)
OFTEN USED WITH Valerian (*Valeriana officinalis*)
CAUTIONS None known. See also pp.42–51.

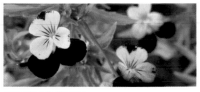

Heartsease, Wild pansy

Viola tricolor

Perhaps appreciated more for its beautiful flowers than as a medicine, heartsease is a valued traditional remedy for skin and chest problems.

MEDICINAL USES

Parts used Aerial parts

Key actions Anti-inflammatory
● Diuretic ● Expectorant

Skin and chest problems Heartease is often combined with herbs such as nettle (*Urtica dioica*) and red clover (*Trifolium pratense*) for skin disorders and to aid detoxification. Commonly used for eczema and other itchy skin conditions, especially in children, heartsease can be taken internally as a tincture or infusion; the latter can be applied to itchy sites. For chest coughs and bronchitis, it combines well with thyme (*Thymus vulgaris*).

FLOWERS AND FOLIAGE

KEY INFORMATION

SAFETY	★ ★ ★ ★ ☆
TRADITIONAL USE	★ ★ ★ ☆ ☆
RESEARCH	★ ☆ ☆ ☆ ☆
BEST TAKEN AS	Infusion ✓✓✓ Tincture ✓✓
DOSAGE	B (*see pp.44–45*)
CAUTION	None known. See also pp.42–51.

Mistletoe

Viscum album

The main therapeutic value of mistletoe lies in treating high blood pressure, although it has traditionally been used to treat epilepsy, insomnia, and tinnitus.

MEDICINAL USES

Parts used Aerial parts (not berries)

Key actions Lowers blood pressure
● Mild sedative

Cardiovascular problems Mildly sedative, mistletoe helps to reduce over-activity, relax blood vessels, and prevent panic attacks. Traditionally thought to act as a heart tonic, mistletoe can prove a useful addition to a formulation for high blood pressure when taken orally. It is best taken after consulting a professional.

KEY INFORMATION

SAFETY	★ ★ ★ ☆ ☆
TRADITIONAL USE	★ ★ ★ ☆ ☆
RESEARCH	★ ★ ☆ ☆ ☆
BEST TAKEN AS	Tincture ✓✓✓ Capsule ✓✓ Tablet ✓
DOSAGE	M, C (*see pp.44–45*)
CAUTIONS	Avoid during pregnancy. Potentially toxic at high dosage. See also pp.42–51.

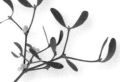

AERIAL PARTS

DRIED STEM

Chaste berry

Vitex agnus-castus

One of the few herbal medicines known to have a progesterone-type activity within the body, chaste berry is a specific for menstrual and perimenopausal problems. Acting on the pituitary gland at the base of the brain, it improves menstrual regularity.

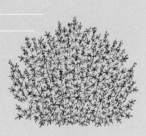

MEDICINAL USES

Part used Fruit

Key actions Hormone balancer
● Stimulates breast milk

Menstrual disorders The essential natural remedy to try in the case of menstrual problems, chaste berry is specifically used to aid in menstrual irregularity and premenstrual syndrome. Though not suitable for all types of menstrual disturbance, it will often help to relieve menstrual symptoms such as breast tenderness, fluid retention, headache, and premenstrual tension. If it is taken over several months, such symptoms will usually become milder and of shorter duration. Tincture or extract is usually taken on awakening in the morning, when the pituitary gland is most active. Chaste berry can be taken to treat heavy menstrual bleeding and period pains, but will work better when combined with other appropriate remedies prescribed by a qualified herbal practitioner.

Polycystic ovary disease Herbal medicine can be

berries have progesterone activity

STEM WITH BERRIES

KEY INFORMATION

SAFETY	★ ★ ★ ★ ☆
TRADITIONAL USE	★ ★ ★ ★ ★
RESEARCH	★ ★ ★ ★ ☆

BEST TAKEN AS Tincture ✓✓✓ Tablet ✓✓ Capsule ✓

DOSAGE M (*see pp.44–45*). Take before breakfast each morning.

OFTEN USED WITH Black cohosh (*Cimicifuga racemosa*)

CAUTION Concurrent use with contraceptive pill, fertility treatment, or hormone replacement therapy is not advisable. Avoid during pregnancy. Rarely, may cause gastrointestinal upset, headache, or dizziness. See also pp.42–51.

tincture is taken for irregular periods

TINCTURE

very helpful in controlling or reversing this difficult problem. Although best treated professionally, self-treatment with chaste berry alone can sometimes bring about a significant improvement in symptoms. It may need to be taken for at least 3–4 months before results are seen.

Infertility Thought to have a pronounced ability to fine tune estrogen and progesterone release through the menstrual cycle, chaste berry can improve fertility and increase the chances of conception. It is most likely to help where there are no structural factors involved.

Menopausal problems Most likely to be of value in the year or so before menopause,

acts on the
pituitary gland

**DRIED
BERRIES**

chaste berry
can help to
maintain a regular
menstrual cycle and control
bleeding. It may also be taken, typically
with remedies such as black cohosh
(*Cimicifuga racemosa*) and sage (*Salvia
officinalis*), to relieve or prevent
menopausal symptoms such as headache,
hot flashes, and night sweats.

Other uses Chaste berry is also used to
treat acne, which is often linked to raised
male hormone levels. Other hormonal
effects include increased breast milk
production in lactating mothers.

MONK'S PEPPER

In medieval times, monks reputedly chewed
chaste berries to curb their sexual desire. In a
similar vein, the 16th-century English herbalist
Gerard wrote: "Agnus castus (or chaste berry) is
a singular medicine for such as
would willingly live chaste, for it
withstandeth all uncleanness or
desire to the flesh,
consuming or drying
up the seed of
generation, in what
sort soever it bee
taken . . . for which
cause it was called
castus, that is to
say chaste, cleane,
and pure."

Chaste berry has a long history of use: Homer
referred it in his epic poem the *Iliad* as a herb
employed to keep all evils at bay.

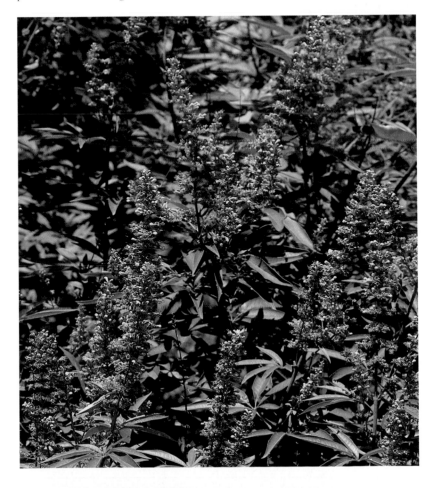

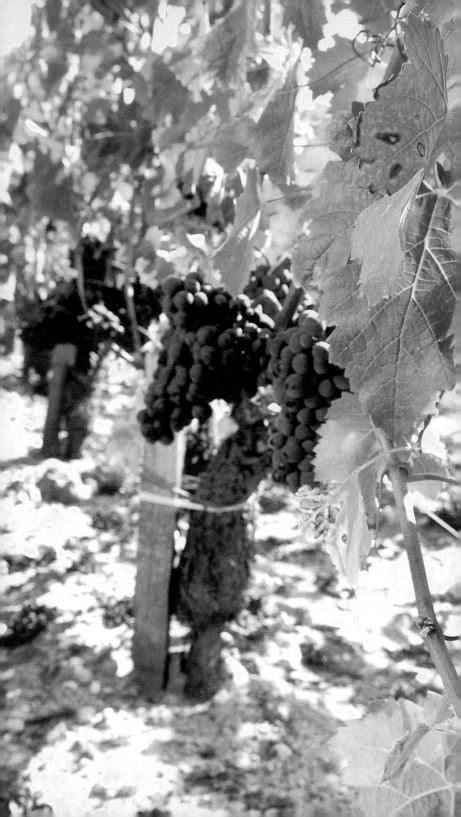

English herbalist Nicholas Culpeper referred to grape vine (*Vitis vinifera*) as "a most gallant tree of the sun very sympathetical to the body of man." Antioxidant and tonic, it has many health benefits.

Grape vine

Vitis vinifera

Grapes have astringent, laxative, and tonic qualities, and are almost universally recommended for convalescence—flowers and grapes are the gifts one brings to the ill and infirm. Traditionally, grapes are used to cool fevers and, as part of a grape fast, promote tissue cleansing.

MEDICINAL USES

Parts used Fresh or dried fruit ● Leaf ● Seed ● Seed oil

Key actions Antioxidant ● Nutritive ● Tonic

Circulatory tonic The beneficial effects of red wine on the heart and circulation are well-known, although red grape juice may be as good if not better. Research has confirmed the antioxidant properties of the red pigments in red grapes. Similar in many respects to the antioxidants in bilberry (*Vaccinium myrtillus*) and maritime pine (*Pinus maritima*), grape seed extract provides powerful antioxidant support to tissues under stress, increasing vitamin C levels within the cells and strengthening blood vessels, particularly small arteries. It is a valuable supplement in chronic conditions affecting the circulation, notably furring up of the arteries (atherosclerosis), peripheral vascular

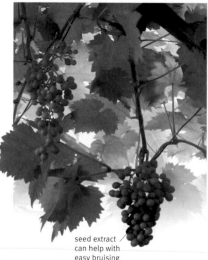

seed extract can help with easy bruising

Native to southern Europe and western Asia, the grape vine is cultivated in warm temperate regions throughout the world for its fruit and to produce wine.

leaves are astringent

GRAPE VINE

disease, including easy bruising, varicose veins, and peripheral neuropathy associated with diabetes.

Sluggish liver and kidneys A grape fast, a naturopathic cleansing regime in which one eats only grapes for several days, helps in detoxifying the body, especially in serious ill health. Although not suitable for everyone, a grape fast can improve health and vitality where liver and kidneys are sluggish. Follow only on professional advice.

Other uses The seeds and leaves are astringent and anti-inflammatory and have been taken to relieve diarrhea. Raisins are highly nutritious, gently laxative, and demulcent.

KEY INFORMATION

SAFETY	★ ★ ★ ★ ★
TRADITIONAL USE	★ ★ ★ ✬ ☆
RESEARCH	★ ★ ★ ✬ ☆
BEST TAKEN AS	Fruit ✓✓✓

Seed extract ✓✓✓ Juice ✓✓
DOSAGE Food; M (*see pp.44–45*)
OFTEN USED WITH Bilberry (*Vaccinium myrtillus*)
CAUTIONS None known. See also pp.42–51.

Withania, Ashwagandha

Withania somniferum

Still relatively unknown in the West, withania has been prized in Ayurvedic medicine for over 4,000 years. Often compared to ginseng, withania is more of a sedative than a stimulant, its calming, restorative action helping to relieve stress and exhaustion.

MEDICINAL USES

Parts used Root • Fruit

Key actions Adaptogen • Sedative • Anti-inflammatory • Tonic

Exhaustion and nervous debility

Withania is a first-rate tonic and building herb, especially useful in conditions involving chronic weakness and nervous debility. It is a good remedy to quiet anxiety states and overactivity and makes an excellent restorative for old age and convalescence. Root and fruit have been used traditionally as a remedy for senile dementia. For best results, the herb should be taken for several months.

Weak immune system Taken long-term, withania strengthens connective tissue

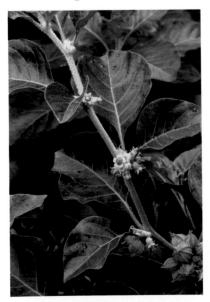

and supports balanced immune function, leading to increased vigor and raised white blood cell count. It therefore has a role to play in a wide range of chronic illnesses, particularly those involving chronic inflammation, such as fibromyalgia and psoriasis. In such conditions it is best taken on professional advice.

Other uses Traditionally valued for its aphrodisiac properties, withania can be taken to improve erectile dysfunction and enhance fertility in men and women. The root and fruit are used in Ayurveda to treat respiratory conditions such as asthma and bronchitis.

KEY INFORMATION

SAFETY	★★★★☆
TRADITIONAL USE	★★★★★
RESEARCH	★★★★☆

BEST TAKEN AS Tablet ✓✓✓ Tincture ✓✓ Decoction ✓

DOSAGE B (*see pp.44–45*)

OFTEN USED WITH Siberian ginseng (*Eleutherococcus senticosus*)

CAUTIONS Avoid during pregnancy. See also pp.42–51.

berries can be taken in convalescence

DRIED BERRIES

root is useful in anemia

FRESH ROOT

This herb is known as "ashwagandha" in Sanskrit, meaning "horse's smell." It also implies a horse's strength, indicative of its use as a strengthening herb.

Prickly ash

Zanthoxylum clava-herculis

A highly valued North American remedy, prickly ash has traditionally been used for numerous conditions, ranging from toothache and rheumatic pain to cramps and poor peripheral circulation. Although bitter and hot to taste, the bark has long been a standby method for cleaning the teeth.

MEDICINAL USES

Parts used Bark ● Fruit

Key actions Analgesic ● Antirheumatic ● Circulatory stimulant ● Stimulates sweating

Rheumatic and arthritic problems By promoting local blood flow and the clearance of waste products, prickly ash can bring relief wherever muscle tension or poor circulation have led to the

FRESH BARK

development of rheumatic symptoms. It can be particularly helpful in relieving chronic musculoskeletal problems such as fibromyalgia. It is generally best combined with anti-inflammatory or antirheumatic remedies, such as meadowsweet (*Filipendula ulmaria*).

Poor peripheral circulation One of the best remedies for

DRIED BERRIES

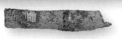

KEY INFORMATION

SAFETY	★★★★☆
TRADITIONAL USE	★★★★☆
RESEARCH	★☆☆☆☆
BEST TAKEN AS	Tincture ✓✓✓
Capsule ✓✓ Tablet ✓	
DOSAGE	C (*see pp.44–45*)
OFTEN USED WITH	Willow bark (*Salix alba*)
CAUTIONS	Avoid during pregnancy and while breast-feeding. See also pp.42–51.

weak circulation, prickly ash is thought to stimulate arterial blood flow. Taken over several weeks or months together with remedies such as cramp bark (*Viburnum opulus*), it can significantly improve peripheral blood flow to the hands and feet. Conditions such as carpal tunnel syndrome, intermittent claudication, Raynaud's disease, varicose veins, and hemorrhoids can all benefit.

Prickly ash bark has a stronger stimulant action on blood flow than the berries, and is normally used when treating peripheral circulatory disorders.

Cornsilk, Maize fronds

Zea mays

Maize is one of the world's most popular foods,
yet few realize that the silky brown fronds wrapped
around the cob make a valuable medicine. Best
prepared as an infusion, cornsilk works specifically
on the urinary system, soothing and protecting the
kidneys, bladder, and urinary tract.

MEDICINAL USES

Part used "Silk" or fronds (pistils)

Key actions Demulcent ● Diuretic
● Mild urinary antiseptic
● Wound healer

Urinary tract problems With diuretic,
demulcent, and mild antiseptic activity,
cornsilk is a remedy to take at the first
sign of urinary infection, helping to
soothe inflammation and irritation
and flush out infection. Protective and
restorative rather than a frontline
treatment for infection, cornsilk supports
kidney function and the health of the
urinary tract. While it is not an effective
treatment on its own, take the infusion
to aid recovery from cystitis and as a
preventative against recurring infection.
The infusion may also help to ease
bladder irritability and poor urine flow.
Use 1 spoonful of chopped cornsilk to a
cup and brew for 15 minutes. Drink up

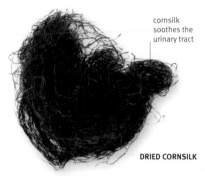

cornsilk
soothes the
urinary tract

DRIED CORNSILK

to 5 cups a day as required. Other
urinary-related problems such as chronic
urethritis and an enlarged prostate can
benefit from this gentle-acting herb. In
cases of kidney disease, including kidney
stones, take only on professional advice.

Other uses Other indications for
cornsilk include high blood pressure and
fluid retention. Despite its diuretic
activity, cornsilk is worth trying in
problems such as stress or pressure
incontinence and bed-wetting.

Ground cornflour mixed to a paste with a little water
makes a good poultice for drawing out a stubborn
and painful splinter.

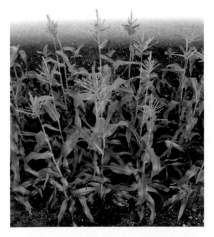

KEY INFORMATION

SAFETY	★ ★ ★ ★ ★
TRADITIONAL USE	★ ★ ★ ★ ☆
RESEARCH	★ ★ ☆ ☆ ☆
BEST TAKEN AS Infusion ✓✓✓	
Tincture ✓✓	

DOSAGE A (*see pp.44–45*)
OFTEN USED WITH Cranberry
(*Vaccinium macrocarpon*)
CAUTIONS None known at normal dosage.
See also pp.42–51.

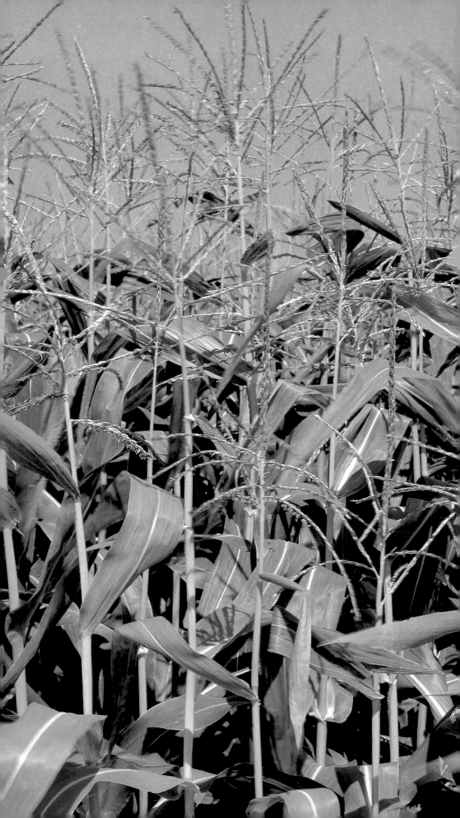

Cultivated for over 4,000 years in Mexico as a food crop, sweetcorn (*Zea mays*) and the silky fronds that surround it are traditionally used to treat kidney and urinary tract disorders.

Ginger

Zingiber officinalis

The warm taste of ginger, one of the most versatile of all spices, adds zest to any herbal infusion. Taken on its own, it stimulates circulation to the skin, promotes sweating and relieves nausea. Combine fresh root with garlic and honey to bring quick relief to colds and flu and settle stomach upset.

MEDICINAL USES

Part used Root (fresh and dry)

Key actions Anti-emetic
- Anti-inflammatory ● Antioxidant
- Circulatory stimulant
- Digestive tonic ● Stimulates sweating

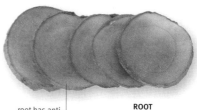

root has anti-inflammatory activity

ROOT

Poor circulation Whether taken on its own or combined with a circulatory stimulant such as ginkgo (*Ginkgo biloba*), ginger helps to tone capillaries and will benefit any condition involving weak or deficient circulation, especially to the head or limbs. Regular intake of ginger—as infusion, tincture or capsule—can make an appreciable difference where poor peripheral circulation is linked to weak digestive function. Ginger has blood-thinning properties so should not be taken at above 2g dried (4g fresh) root by those taking anticoagulants.

Nausea and vomiting Probably ginger's most valuable area of activity, supported by in-depth research, is as a safe and effective remedy for nausea, vomiting, motion sickness, and morning sickness during pregnancy. Take ginger tea or a standardized extract at the earliest signs of symptoms. If using for travel sickness, start taking the tea or extract before

Pungent and somewhat lemony in taste, ginger has a multitude of uses that have gained it the label of "the best medicine in the world."

KEY INFORMATION

SAFETY   ★ ★ ★ ★ ✩
TRADITIONAL USE   ★ ★ ★ ★ ★
RESEARCH   ★ ★ ★ ✩ ☆
BEST TAKEN AS Infusion ✓✓✓
Capsule ✓✓ Tincture ✓
DOSAGE Fresh root: C ; Dried root: D (*see pp.44–45*)
OFTEN USED WITH Garlic (*Allium sativum*)
CAUTIONS Maximum dose during pregnancy and if taking anticoagulants is 2g dried (4g fresh) root a day. Can cause discomfort in stomach disorders. See also pp.42–51.

beginning your journey. Ginger also makes a good remedy for symptoms such as intestinal colic, gas, and bloating. An underappreciated remedy for gastro-intestinal infection, it can provide significant relief in symptoms such as indigestion, bloating, and diarrhea.

Anti-inflammatory action Recent research has shown ginger root to have potent anti-inflammatory activity, making it a possible alternative to aspirin-type medicines in treating arthritic pain. As relatively large doses are required, seek professional advice in this situation.

Viral infection When a cold, flu, cough, or chest infection threatens, fresh ginger root tea can improve resistance as well as one's sense of well-being. The tea combines well with other remedies such as cinnamon, garlic, and licorice.

DIGESTIVE REMEDY

Ginger's positive effects on the dige are the subject of ongoing scientific s Several clinical trials have shown that g extract relieves post-operative nausea an vomiting, with a low incidence of side effec Evidence also supports ginger's use in reliev travel sickness, as well as nausea and vomiting during pregnancy. Active constituents in ginger are thought to stimulate stomach activity and to relieve spasm, which also helps in gastrointestinal disorders such as cramps, colic, and diarrhea.

CAPSULES

Other uses

Ginger is included in numerous herbal formulations and can, where indicated, be combined with almost any other remedy. Some of the many conditions that it can benefit include: period pain (take symptomatically with remedies such as cramp bark (*Viburnum opulus*); irregular menstrual cycle; anemia and lowered vitality, where it combines well with *Withania somnifera*; and headache and migraine. Evidence also points to ginger root lowering cholesterol levels and protecting against stomach ulcers.

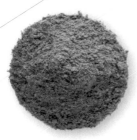

POWDER

FRESH SHOOT

root stimulat s periphera circulation

root has antiviral properties

FRESH ROOT

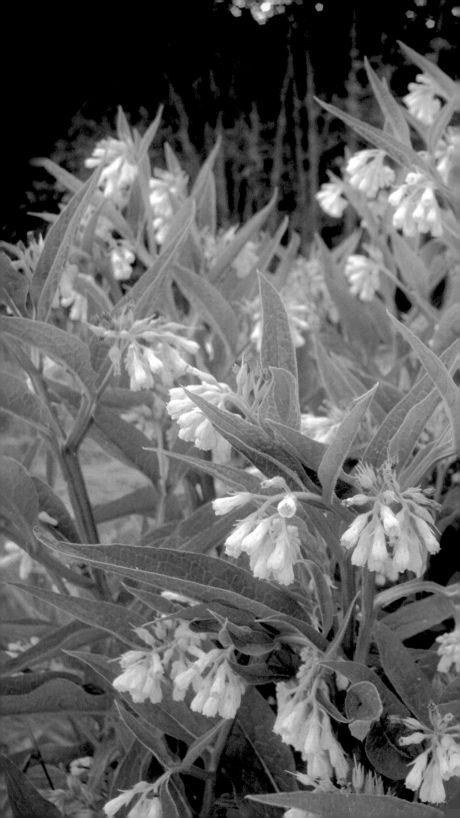

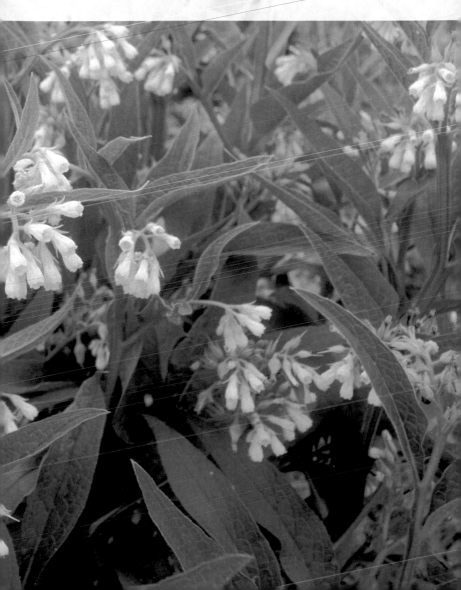

COMMON
HEALTH
PROBLEMS

REMEDIES FOR HOME USE

The following section gives straightforward recommendations for remedies that can be safely used at home to treat many common health problems. A number of remedies are suggested for each condition, and these can be used individually or in combination.

How to use this section

GENERAL GUIDELINES

1. Be clear about what condition it is that needs treating. If you are unsure, seek professional advice, such as a telephone help line.
2. Select the herb(s) you wish to use from the list and look up in A–Z of Herbal Remedies, pp.52–255. Note the dosage and cautions listed in key information box (*see also p.45*)
3. Decide how to take the herb(s), for example as an infusion.
4. Work out an appropriate dosage (*see also pp.44–45*): Take a single remedy as recommended; for combined remedies, work out which herb has the lowest recommended dosage and

take the combination at this dosage. Medium to high doses can be taken for up to 4 days; lower doses are required when taking an herbal remedy longer term.
5. Teas and decoctions: the dosages given apply when making teas and decoctions from dried herb material—bark, leaves, roots, etc. For fresh herb material you can use 1 ½– 2 times the quantity of dried material.
6. Tinctures: It is not possible to give clear guidelines for tinctures owing to the wide variation in their strength. Ask advice on dosage when purchasing a tincture. In general, the dosage range for a 1:3 tincture is the same (in millilitres not grams) as the dosages in the Recommended adult dosage box (*left*), i.e. for A, the dosage of a 1:3 tincture is 5–15ml a day.
7. Powders: take the minimum recommended daily dosage only.
8. Tablets and capsules: Take at the manufacturer's recommended dosage.

RECOMMENDED ADULT DOSAGE

See also pp.44–45. If over-70, see p.45. For children, see pp.44, 47, and 273–275. Look up the dosage for each remedy.

A   5–15g a day, or max. 100g (3½ oz) per week

B   3–7.5g a day, or max. 50g (2 oz) per week

C   2–4g a day, or max. 30g (1 oz) per week

D   1–2g a day, or max 15g (½ oz) per week

M   Take product at manufacturer's recommended dosage

T   Topical application on the skin only (not to be taken internally)

KEY TO PAGES 259–275

T   TEA OR INFUSION (*pp.31, 34*)

D   DECOCTION (*pp.31, 34*)

Tr   TINCTURE (*pp.32, 35*)

C   CAPSULE OR TABLET (*p.32*)

S   SYRUP (*p.32*)

G   GARGLE

EO   ESSENTIAL OIL, external use only (*p.33*)

L   LOCAL USE, cream, ointment, lotion; other application in brackets (*p.33*)

HEAD

CONDITION	HERB	PREPARATION
Tension headache	Limeflower (pp.224–225)	T, Tr, C
	Lavender (pp.152–153)	L (EO)
	Skullcap (p.205)	T, Tr, C
	Guarana (p.172)	T, C
Migraine	Feverfew (p.213)	Tr, C
	Butterbur (p.178)	C
	Lavender (pp.152–153)	L (EO)
Menstrual headache	Chaste berry (pp.244–245)	Tr, C
	Skullcap (p.205)	T, Tr, C
	Feverfew (p.213)	Tr, C
Dizziness	Black cohosh (pp.100–101)	Tr
	Ginkgo (pp.138–139)	Tr, C
	Rosemary (p.190)	T, Tr, C
Tinnitus	Ginkgo (pp.138–139)	Tr, C
	Mistletoe (p.243)	Tr, C
	Black cohosh (pp.100–101)	Tr, C
Earache	Garlic (pp.60–61)	L (O)
	Elderflower (pp.202–203)	T, Tr, C, S
	Goldenseal (p.147)	Tr, C
	Lavender (pp.152–153)	L (EO)
Infection of ears, sinuses, and nose	Elderberry (p.202)	S Tr, C
	Echinacea (pp.118–119)	T, Tr, C
	Andrographis (p.55)	Tr, C
	Thyme (p.222)	T, Tr, C
Catarrh and congestion	Elderflower (pp.202–203)	T, Tr, C
	Plantain (p.181)	T, Tr, C
	Goldenseal (p.147)	Tr, C
	Sage (p.200)	T, Tr, C
Hay fever and allergy	Eyebright (p.129)	T, Tr, C
	Baical skullcap (p.204)	T, Tr, C
	Butterbur (p.178)	C
	Eldeflower (pp.202–203)	T, Tr, C
Nosebleed	Yarrow (p.54)	T, Tr, C
	Nettle (pp.234–235)	T, Tr, C
	Golden seal (p.147)	Tr, C

HEAD (CONTINUED)

CONDITION	HERB	PREPARATION
Sties	Calendula (p.86)	L (ointment)
	Chamomile (pp.98–99)	L (lotion)
	Goldenseal (p.147)	L (ointment)
Conjunctivitis	Eyebright (p.129)	L (lotion) T, Tr, C
	Echinacea (pp.118–119)	T, Tr, C
	Witch hazel (p.144)	L (distilled water)
Sore eyes/lids	Witch hazel (p.144)	L (distilled water)
	Chamomile (pp.98–99)	L (T)
Poor eyesight	Bilberry (p.237)	T, Tr, C S
	Ginkgo (pp.138–139)	Tr, C
	Eyebright (p.129)	T, Tr, C
Toothache	Clove (pp.37, 123)	L (1 clove or 1 drop EO)
Dental treatment	St. John's wort (pp.148–149)	L (oil)
Mouth ulcers	Myrrh (p.107)	L (diluted Tr)
	Licorice (pp.140–141)	L (neat Tr)
	Echinacea (pp.118–119)	L (diluted Tr)
Gum problems	Bilberry (p.237)	L (T or Tr)
	Myrrh (p.107)	L (diluted Tr)
	Yarrow (p.54)	L (T or Tr)
Thrush (mouth)	Cat's claw (p.233)	Tr, C, L (diluted Tr)
	Pau d'arco (p.214)	Tr, C, L (diluted Tr)

CAUTIONS FOR HEAD CONDITIONS

Seek immediate professional advice for:
- Fever of 102°F (39°C) or above
- Heavy nosebleed lasting more than 1 hour
- Persistent one-sided headache
- Headache or pain that fails to improve within 48 hours despite self-medication
- Double vision/visual disturbance
- Unexplained dizziness
- Sudden or severe allergy

THROAT, CHEST, AND LUNGS

CONDITION	HERB	PREPARATION
Colds, flu colds	Ginger (pp.254–255)	T, Tr, C
	Andrographis (p.55)	Tr, C
	Echinacea (pp.118–119)	T, Tr, C
	Cinnamon (p.97)	T, Tr, C
	Yarrow (p.54)	T, Tr
	Elderflower/berry (pp.202–203)	T, Tr, S
Sore throat/hoarseness	Sage (p.200)	G T, Tr
	Echinacea (pp.118–119)	G T, Tr
	Plantain (p.181)	G T, Tr
Catarrh and congestion	Elderflower (pp.202–203)	T, Tr, C
	Thyme (p.222)	T, Tr, C
	Elecampane (p.150)	T, Tr, C
	Garlic (pp.60–61)	C, or with food
Cough	Thyme (p.222)	T, Tr, C
	Licorice (pp.140–141)	T, Tr, C
	Elecampane (p.150)	T, Tr, C
	Caraway (p.94)	T, Tr, C
Shortness of breath	Baical skullcap (p.204)	T, Tr, C
	Angelica (p.67)	T, Tr, C
	Thyme (p.222)	T, Tr, C
	Lobelia (p.157)	C
Bronchitis	Elecampane (p.150)	T, Tr, C
	Thyme (p.222)	T, Tr, C
	Caraway (p.94)	T, Tr, C
	Lobelia (p.157)	C
Preventing infection	Elderberry (p.202)	T, Tr, S C
	Sea buckthorn (p.146)	T, S, C
	Thyme (p.222)	T, Tr, C
	Echinacea (pp.118–119)	T, Tr, C

CAUTIONS FOR THROAT, CHEST, AND LUNG CONDITIONS

Seek immediate professional advice for:
• Fever of 102°F (39°C) or above
• Allergic reactions, including asthma
• Allergies that worsen after taking herbal remedies
• Persistent hoarseness, cough, or sore throat
• Chest pain or shortness of breath
• Coughing up blood

DIGESTION

CONDITION	HERB	PREPARATION
Poor appetite	Gentian (p.136)	Tr,
	Alfalfa (p.162)	Tr, C
	Angelica (p.67)	Tr
Acid indigestion/reflux	Meadowsweet (p.130)	T, Tr
	Marshmallow (p.66)	T, Tr
	Licorice (pp.140–141)	T, Tr
	Chamomile (pp.98–99)	T, Tr
Nausea/motion sickness	Ginger (pp.254–255)	T, Tr, C
	Chamomile (pp.98–99)	T, Tr, C
	Lemon balm (p.164)	T, Tr,
Indigestion, gas, and bloating	Fennel (pp.131)	T, Tr, C
	Cardamon (p.122)	T, Tr, C
	Peppermint (p.165)	T, Tr, C
	Oregano (p.171)	T, Tr, C
Digestive infections	Garlic (pp.60–61)	C, or with food
	Cat's claw (p.233)	Tr, C
	Goldenseal (p.147)	Tr, C
	Calendula (p.86)	T, Tr, C
	Cinnamon (p.97)	T, Tr, C
Worms	Pumpkin seeds (p.109)	Ground seeds
	Thyme (p.222)	T, Tr, C
	Garlic (pp.60–61)	C, or with food
Cramps and pain	Cramp bark (p.242)	T, Tr, C
	Chamomile (pp.98–99)	T, Tr, C
	Ginger (pp.254–255)	T, Tr, C
Diarrhea	Plantain (p.181)	T, Tr, C
	Slippery elm (p.232)	T, C
	Raspberry leaf (p.191)	T, Tr, C
Constipation	Flaxseed (p.158–159)	T
	Rhubarb root (p.185)	Tr, C
	Senna (p.87)	T, C
Irritable bowel	Peppermint (p.165)	T, Tr, C
	Valerian (p.240)	T, Tr, C
	Clove (p.123)	T, Tr, C
	Aloe vera (pp.62–63)	Juice or C

DIGESTION (CONTINUED)		
CONDITION	HERB	PREPARATION
Supporting liver/ gall-bladder	Milk thistle (p.207)	C
	Dandelion (p.215)	T, Tr, C
	Bupleurum (p.83)	C Tr
	Schisandra (p.201)	T, Tr, C
Helping weight loss	Kelp (p.134)	C Tr
	Globe artichoke (pp.113)	C Tr
Helping weight gain	Alfalfa (p.162)	T, or as food
	Fenugreek	T, C, or as food

CAUTIONS FOR DIGESTIVE CONDITIONS

Seek immediate professional advice for:
- Difficulty in swallowing
- Persistent abdominal pain or indigestion
- Change in bowel habit
- Passing blood in the stool
- Persistent weight loss

CIRCULATION AND HEART

CONDITION	HERB	PREPARATION
High blood pressure	Hawthorn (pp.110–111)	C Tr, T,
	Dan shen (p.197)	T, Tr, C
	Dandelion leaf (p.215)	T, Tr, C
	Yarrow (p.54)	T, Tr, C
Low blood pressure	Rosemary (p.190)	T, Tr, C
	Licorice (pp.140–141)	Tr, C
	Nettle leaf (pp.234–235)	T, Tr, C
Palpitations	Motherwort (p.156)	T, Tr, C
	Limeflower (pp.224–225)	T, Tr, C
	Lemon Balm (p.164)	T, Tr, C
Poor peripheral circulation	Ginkgo (pp.138–139)	Tr, C
	Cinnamon (p.97)	T, Tr, C
	Cayenne pepper (pp.90–91)	C

CIRCULATION AND HEART (CONTINUED)

CONDITION	HERB	PREPARATION
Varicose veins/ hemorrhoids	Horse chestnut (pp.56–57)	C, Tr
	Butcher's broom (p.194)	C, Tr
	Witch hazel (p.144)	L (distilled water)
	Gotu kola (p.95)	Tr, C
	Bilberry (p.237)	T, Tr, C
Poor healing	Gotu kola (p.95)	Tr, C
	Yarrow (p.54)	T, Tr, C
	Plantain (p.181)	T, Tr, C
	Comfrey (pp.211)	L
Supporting heart and circulation	Hawthorn (pp.110–111)	C, Tr, T
	Motherwort (p.156)	T, Tr, C
	Garlic (pp.60–61)	C, or with food

CAUTIONS FOR CIRCULATION AND HEART CONDITIONS

Seek immediate professional advice for:
• Chest pain or shortness of breath
• Unexplained dizziness
• Hot, swollen, or ulcerated tender veins

BLOOD, METABOLIC

CONDITION	HERB	PREPARATION
Anemia	Nettle (pp.234–235)	T, Tr, C
	Parsley leaf (p.179)	T, or as food
	Gentian (p.136)	Tr
Raised cholesterol levels	Guggul (p.107)	C
	Turmeric (p.112)	C
	Alfalfa (p.162)	T, or as food
	Globe artichoke (p.113)	C
Unstable bloodsugar levels	Holy basil (p.167)	T, Tr, C
	Gymnema (p.136)	Tr, C
	Cinnamon (p.97)	T, Tr, C

BLOOD, METABOLIC (CONTINUED)

CONDITION	HERB	PREPARATION
Overactive thyroid	Motherwort (p.156)	T, Tr, C
	Lemon balm (p.164)	T, Tr, C
	Withania (p.249)	Tr, C
Underactive thyroid	Kelp (p.134)	C
	Cayenne pepper (pp.90–91)	C
	Siberian ginseng (p.124–125)	Tr, C

CAUTIONS FOR BLOOD, METABOLIC CONDITIONS

Seek immediate professional advice for:
- Persistent weight loss
- Frequent and excessive urination

BLADDER AND URINARY TRACT

CONDITION	HERB	PREPARATION
Cystitis	Cranberry (p.236)	Juice, Tr, C
	Buchu (p.80)	T, Tr, C
	Crataeva (p.108)	T, Tr, C
	Cornsilk (p.251)	T, Tr, C
Urethritis	Cranberry (p.236)	Juice, Tr, C
	Cornsilk (p.251)	T, Tr, C
	Puncture vine (p.223)	Tr, C
Frequency	Cornsilk (p.251)	T, Tr, C
	Cramp bark (p.242)	T, Tr, C
	Passion flower (p.173)	T, Tr, C

CAUTIONS FOR BLADDER AND URINARY TRACT CONDITIONS

Seek immediate professional advice for:
- Passing blood in the urine
- Pain in the kidneys
- Fever of 102°F (39°C) or above
- Urinary infections that deteriorate despite taking herbal remedies

JOINTS, MUSCLES, AND BONE

CONDITION	HERB	PREPARATION
Sprains, bruises, and sports injuries	Comfrey (p.211) Arnica (p.66) Gotu kola (p.95)	L L Tr, C
Fractures	Comfrey (p.211) Plantain (p.181) Yarrow (p.54)	L L, Tr, C L, Tr, C
Muscular aches and pains	Birch (p.81) Prickly ash (p.250) Bogbean (p.166) Meadowsweet (p.130)	T, Tr, C Tr, C Tr, C T, Tr, C
Joint pain and stiffness	Devil's claw (p.145) Boswellia (p.82) Willow bark (p.196) Celery seed (p.69)	C, Tr C C, Tr C, Tr
Chronic inflammation	Boswellia (p.82) Willow bark (p.196) Golden root (p.186) Turmeric (p.112)	C C, Tr C, Tr C, Tr
Back problems	Cramp bark (p.242) St. John's wort (pp.148–149) Prickly ash (p.250) Boswellia (p.82)	Tr, C T, Tr, C, L (oil) Tr, C C
Restless legs	Cramp bark (p.242) Chamomile (pp.98–99) Prickly ash (p.250) Lavender (pp.152–153)	Tr, C T, Tr, C Tr, C L (EO)
Supporting muscular-skeletal health as food	Alfalfa (p.162) Flaxseed (pp.158–159) Meadowsweet (p.130)	T, or as food Ground seed T, Tr, C

CAUTIONS FOR JOINT, MUSCLE, AND BONE CONDITIONS

Seek immediate professional advice for:
- Frequent and persistent back pain
- Unexplained leg pain and swelling
- Broken or suspected broken bones
- Any injury that may need an X-ray

SKIN

CONDITION	HERB	PREPARATION
Acne and boils	Burdock (p.72)	D, Tr, C
	Yellow dock (p.195)	D, Tr, C
	Red clover (pp.226–227)	T, Tr, C
	Echinacea (pp.118–119)	T, Tr, C
	Tea tree (p.163)	L (EO)
Nettle rash	Nettle leaf (pp.234–235)	T, Tr, C
	Baical skullcap (p.204)	T, Tr, C
	Chamomile (pp.98–99)	T, Tr, C
	Aloe vera (pp.62–63)	L (juice/gel)
Itchiness	Chickweed (p.212)	L
	Witch hazel (p.144)	L
	Evening primrose oil (p.170)	L
	Borage oil (p.80)	L
Eczema	Oregon grape (p.77)	D, Tr, C
	Calendula (p.86)	T, Tr, C
	Burdock (p.72)	D, Tr, C
	Gotu kola (p.95)	T, Tr, C
Fungal infections	Golden seal (p.147)	Tr, C
	Echinacea (pp.118–119)	Tr, C
	Thyme (p.222)	T, Tr, C
	Tea tree (p.163)	L (EO)
Herpes sores/shingles	Echinacea (pp.118–119)	Tr, C
	Passion flower (p.173)	T, Tr, C
	St. John's wort (pp.148–149)	T, Tr, C
	Pau d'arco (p.214)	D, Tr, C
Warts	Thuja (p.219)	Tr
	Garlic (pp.60–61)	L
Cuts, grazes, and minor wounds	Calendula (p.86)	L
	Aloe vera (pp.62–63)	Juice/gel
	Yarrow (p.54)	L
Bruises	Arnica (p.66)	L
	Comfrey (p.211)	L
	Plantain (p.181)	T, Tr, C, L
	Gotu kola (p.95)	T, Tr, C, L

SKIN

CONDITION	HERB	PREPARATION
Minor burns	Aloe vera (pp.62–63)	Juice/gel
	Calendula (p.86)	L (lotion or cream)
	St. John's wort (pp.148–149)	L (oil)
	Witch hazel (p.144)	L (distilled water)
Sunburn	Aloe vera (pp.62–63)	Juice/gel
	Calendula (p.86)	L
Headlice	Neem (p.75)	L
Detox/supporting skin health	Dandelion root (p.215)	D, Tr, C
	Nettle (pp.234–235)	T, Tr, C
	Red clover (pp.226–227)	T, Tr, C
	Yellow dock (p.195)	D, Tr, C

CAUTIONS FOR SKIN PROBLEMS

Seek immediate professional advice for:
- Serious wounds, grazes, bruising, bites, and stings
- Sudden swelling or allergic reaction
- Non-minor burns, including sunburn
- A mole that has changed shape, size or color, or itches or bleeds
- A sore or boil that does not heal, or unexplained swellings under the skin
- Shingles or suspected shingles

WOMEN'S HEALTH PROBLEMS

CONDITION	HERB	PREPARATION
Premenstrual tension	Chaste berry (pp.244–245)	Tr, C
	Black cohosh (pp.100–101)	Tr, C
	Skullcap (p.205)	T, Tr, C
	Evening primrose oil (p.170)	C
Pain/cramps	Cramp bark (p.242)	T, Tr, C
	White peony (p.172)	T, Tr, C
	Skullcap (p.205)	T, Tr, C
	Motherwort (p.156)	T, Tr, C
Heavy bleeding	Raspberry leaf (p.191)	T, Tr, C
	Nettle (pp.234–235)	T, Tr, C
	Yarrow (p.54)	T, Tr, C

WOMEN'S HEALTH PROBLEMS (CONTINUED)

CONDITION	HERB	PREPARATION
Scant bleeding	Chinese angelica (p.68)	D, Tr, C
	White peony (p.172)	T, Tr, C
	Black cohosh (pp.100–101)	Tr, C
	Motherwort (p.156)	T, Tr, C
Irregular cycle	Chaste berry (pp.244–245)	Tr, C
	White peony (p.172)	T, Tr, C
	Black cohosh (pp.100–101)	Tr, C
Helping fertility	Chaste berry (pp.244–245)	Tr, C
	Motherwort (p.156)	T, Tr, C
Sore breasts	Calendula (pp.84–85, 86)	T, Tr, C
	Red clover (pp.226–227)	T, Tr, C
	Echinacea (p.118–119)	T, Tr, C
Thrush	Cat's claw (p.233)	Tr, C
	Oregano (p.171)	T, Tr, C
	Tea tree (p.163)	L (pessary)
Menopausal problems	Black cohosh (pp.100–101)	Tr, C
	Sage (p.200)	T (cooled), Tr, C
	Alfalfa (p.162)	C, or as food
	Puncture vine (p.223)	Tr, C
	Licorice (pp.140–141)	Tr, C
	Wild yam (pp.116–117)	Tr, C
Osteoporosis	Black cohosh (pp.100–101)	Tr, C
	Withania (p.249)	Tr, C
	Alfalfa (p.162)	T, C, or as food

CAUTIONS FOR WOMEN'S HEALTH PROBLEMS

Seek immediate professional advice for:
- Persistent pain in abdomen or pelvis
- Vaginal bleeding between periods, after sex, or following menopause
- Any unusual vaginal discharge
- Thickening, lump or change in shape in a breast
- Discharge from a nipple

PREGNANCY

CONDITION	HERB	PREPARATION
Morning sickness	Ginger (pp.254–255)	T, C
	Chamomile (pp.98–99)	T, C
	Slippery elm (p.232)	T
Constipation	Flaxseed (pp.158–159)	Food
	Dandelion root (p.215)	D, C
	Senna (p.87)	C
Varicose veins/hemorrhoids	Witch hazel (p.144)	L (distilled water)
Colds, flu colds	Elderflower/berry (pp.202–203)	T, S, C
	Sea buckthorn (p.146)	T, S, C
	Echinacea (pp.118–119)	T, C
	Plantain (p.181)	T, C
Poor sleep	Passion flower (p.173)	T, C
	Valerian (p.240)	T, C
	Skullcap (p.205)	T, C
	Lemon balm (p.164)	T

CAUTIONS FOR PREGNANCY

Seek immediate professional advice for:
• Prolonged nausea causing inability to eat
• Frequent vomiting
• Frequent urination for more than 3 days
• Breast pain with swollen glands under the arms or a fever
• Fluid retention that has not reduced after 3 days
See also: Pregnancy and after, pp.46–47

MEN'S HEALTH PROBLEMS

CONDITION	HERB	PREPARATION
Erectile dysfunction	Ginseng (pp.176–177)	Tr, C
	Ginkgo (pp.138–139)	Tr, C
	Saw palmetto (p.206)	C
	Puncture vine (p.223)	Tr, C
Infertility	Pumpkin seeds (p.109)	Food
	Ginseng (pp.176–177)	Tr, C
	Golden root (p.186)	Tr, C

MEN'S HEALTH PROBLEMS (CONTINUED)

CONDITION	HERB	PREPARATION
Prostate probems	Saw palmetto (p.206)	C
	Nettle root (pp.234–235)	C
	Pumpkin seeds (p.109)	Food

CAUTIONS FOR MEN'S HEALTH PROBLEMS

Seek immediate professional advice for:
- swelling or lump in the testicle
- change in shape or size of the testicle
- total and persistent failure to get an erection

MENTAL AND EMOTIONAL PROBLEMS

CONDITION	HERB	PREPARATION
Anxiety/nervousness	Valerian (p.240)	D, Tr, C
	Lemon balm (p.164)	T, Tr, C
	Limeflowers (pp.224–225)	T, Tr, C
	Motherwort (p.156)	T, Tr, C
Depressed mood	St. John's Wort (pp.148–149)	Tr, C
	Damiana (p.231)	T, Tr, C
	Golden root (p.186)	Tr, C
	Rosemary (p.190)	T, Tr, C
Chronic stress	Siberian ginseng (pp.124–125)	Tr, C
	Ginseng (pp.176–177)	Tr, C
	Withania (p.249)	Tr, C
	Licorice (pp.140–141)	T, Tr, C
SAD (Winter "blues")	St. John's Wort (pp.148–149)	Tr, C
	Golden root (p.186)	Tr, C
	Rosemary (p.190)	T, Tr, C
Difficulty in sleeping	Passion flower (p.173)	T, Tr, C
	Valerian (p.240)	D, Tr, C
	Californian poppy (p.128)	T, Tr, C
	Hops (p.147)	Tr, C
Nervous exhaustion	Skullcap (p.205)	T, Tr, C
	Vervain (p.241)	T, Tr, C
	Oats (p.74)	T, Tr, C
	Siberian ginseng (pp.124–125)	Tr, C

MENTAL AND EMOTIONAL PROBLEMS (CONTINUED)

CONDITION	HERB	PREPARATION
Poor memory/ concentration	Ginkgo (pp.138–139)	Tr, C
	Rosemary (p.190)	T, Tr, C
	Sage (p.200)	T, Tr, C
	Schisandra (p.201)	T, Tr, C

CAUTIONS FOR MENTAL AND EMOTIONAL PROBLEMS

Seek professional help and advice for persistent or severe emotional and nervous problems.

PROMOTING HEALTH AND PERFORMANCE

CONDITION	HERB	PREPARATION
Physical stamina	Ginseng (pp.176–177)	Tr, C
	Siberian ginseng (pp.124–125)	Tr, C
	Golden root (p.186)	Tr, C
	Ginkgo (pp.138–139)	Tr, C
Exams	Rosemary (p.190)	T, Tr, C
	Ginkgo (pp.138–139)	Tr, C
	Siberian ginseng (pp.124–125)	Tr, C
	Schisandra (p.201)	T, Tr, C

SUPPORTING IMMUNE FUNCTION

CONDITION	HERB	PREPARATION
Chronic infection	Astragalus (p.73)	Tr, C
	Echinacea (pp.118–119)	Tr, C
	Cat's claw (p.233)	Tr, C
	Siberian ginseng (pp.124–125)	Tr, C
Depleted immune system	Reishi (p.135)	C
	Shiitake (p.151)	C, or as food
	Astragalus (p.73)	Tr, C
	Golden root (p.186)	Tr, C

Children's common health problems

The following are recommendations specifically for the home treatment of children between 6 months and 12 years of age. The herbal remedies selected are considered safe for children between these ages. For babies up to 6 months, seek professional advice before giving them a herbal remedy.

Common health problems, as listed below, can be safely treated with herbal remedies. For other conditions, seek advice from your herbal or medical practitioner.

If your child is showing any of the signs listed under the Cautions, seek immediate medical advice and treatment. In children, potentially serious illness needs to be treated as quickly as possible. If in doubt, always err on the side of caution and seek advice.

DOSAGE LEVELS FOR CHILDREN

NB Do not give babies under 6 months herbal remedies without professional advice. You may need to adjust dosage levels for children who are particularly small or large for their age.

From 6 months to 1 year
$1/10$ minimum adult dose

From 1 to 6 years
$1/3$ minimum adult dose

From 7 to 11 years
$1/2$ minimum adult dose

From 12 to 16 years
Low adult dose

See also general advice on pp.44–45 and on p.47.

HEAD AND CHEST

CONDITION	HERB	PREPARATION
Tension headache and migraine	Limeflower (pp.224–225)	T, Tr, C
	Lemon balm (p.164)	T, Tr, C
	Lavender (pp.152–153)	L (diluted EO)
Earache	Garlic (pp.60–61)	L (O), C
	Elderflower (pp.202–203)	T, Tr, C, S
	Lavender (pp.152–153)	L (diluted EO)
Sties	Calendula (p.86)	L (ointment)
	Goldenseal (p.147)	L (ointment)
Conjunctivitis	Eyebright (p.129)	L (lotion), T Tr, C
	Echinacea (pp.118–119)	T, Tr, C
	Witch hazel (p.144)	L (distilled water)
Sore eyes/lids	Witch hazel (p.144)	L (distilled water)
	Chamomile (pp.98–99)	L (T)
Toothache	Clove (p.123)	L (1 clove or 1 drop EO)

HEAD AND CHEST (CONTINUED)

CONDITION	HERB	PREPARATION
Mouth ulcers/oral thrush	Licorice (pp.140–141)	L, (neat, Tr)
	Echinacea (pp.118–119)	L (diluted Tr)
Nosebleed	Nettle (pp.234–235)	T, Tr, C
Hay fever and allergy	Eyebright (p.129)	T, Tr, C
	Baical skullcap (p.204)	T, Tr, C
	Elderflower (pp.202–203)	T, Tr, C
Feverish states	Elderflower (p.202–203)	T
	Meadowsweet (p.130)	T
	Limeflowers (p.224–225)	T
Colds, flu colds	Elderflower/berry (pp.202–203)	T, Tr, S
	Echinacea (pp.118–119)	T, Tr, C
	Cinnamon (p.97)	T, Tr, C
	Thyme (p.222)	T, Tr, C, S
Sore throat	Echinacea (pp.118–119)	G T, Tr
	Plantain (p.181)	G T, Tr
	Licorice (pp.140–141)	G T, Tr
Cough, catarrh, and congestion	Elderflower (pp.202–203)	T, Tr, C
	Thyme (p.222)	T, Tr, C
	Garlic (pp.60–61)	C, or with food
Preventing infection	Elderberry (pp.202–203)	T, Tr, S
	Sea buckthorn (p.146)	S
	Blackcurrant	Juice, S

CAUTIONS FOR HEAD AND CHEST CONDITIONS

Seek immediate professional advice for:
- Fever of 102°F (39°C) or above
- Heavy nosebleed lasting more than 1 hour
- Persistent one-sided headache or headache or pain that fails to improve within 48 hours despite over-the-counter medication
- Double vision/visual disturbance
- Unexplained dizziness
- Sudden or severe allergy
- Allergic reactions, including asthma
- Allergies that worsen after taking herbal remedies
- Persistent hoarseness, cough, or sore throat
- Chest pain or shortness of breath
- Coughing up blood

DIGESTION

CONDITION	HERB	PREPARATION
Poor appetite	Dandelion root (p.215)	Tr
	Alfalfa (p.162)	T, or as food
Stomach ache	Meadowsweet (p.130)	T, T
	Marshmallow (p.66)	T, Tr
	Chamomile (pp.98–99)	T, Tr
Nausea/motion sickness	Ginger (pp.254–255)	T, C
	Chamomile (pp.98–99)	T, Tr, C
Indigestion, gas, and bloating	Fennel (p.131)	T, Tr, C
	Caraway (p.94)	T, Tr, C
Digestive infections	Garlic (pp.60–61)	C, or with food
	Echinacea (pp.118–119)	Tr, C
	Cinnamon (p.97)	T, Tr, C
Worms	Pumpkin seeds (p.109)	Ground seeds
	Thyme (p.222)	T, Tr, C
	Garlic (pp.60–61)	C, or with food
Cramps and pain	Cramp bark (p.242)	T, Tr, C
	Chamomile (pp.98–99)	T, Tr, C
	Ginger (pp.60–61)	T, C
Diarrhea	Plantain (p.181)	T, Tr, C
	Raspberry leaf (p.191)	T, Tr, C
	Slippery elm (p.232)	T, C
Constipation	Flaxseed (pp.158–159)	T
	Slippery elm (p.232)	T

CAUTIONS FOR DIGESTIVE CONDITIONS

Seek immediate professional advice for:
- Difficulty in swallowing
- Persistent abdominal pain or indigestion
- Passing blood in the stool
- Weight loss or failure to thrive

Glossary

A

Adaptogen Aids the body in adapting to stress, supports healthy function

Aerial parts Above-ground parts of the plant

Analgesic Reduces or relieves pain

Antibacterial Combats bacterial infection

Antibiotic Destroys or inhibits micro-organisms

Anticatarrhal Reduces or relieves catarrh and congestion

Anticoagulant Prevents blood clotting, thins the blood

Antiemetic Reduces or relives nausea and sickness

Antifungal Combats fungal infection

Antihemorrhagic Reduces or stops bleeding

Anti-inflammatory Reduces inflammation

Antioxidant Prevents oxidation and breakdown of tissues

Antiseptic Destroys or inhibits micro-organisms that cause infection

Antispasmodic Relieves muscle cramps or reduces muscle tone

Antiviral Combats viral infection

Aphrodisiac Excites libido and the sexual organs

Aromatic Having an aroma

Astringent Tightens mucous membranes and skin, reducing secretions and bleeding from abrasions

Autoimmune Acute or chronic illness caused by immune system attacking itself

Ayurveda Traditional Indian and Sri Lankan system of medicine

B

Bitter Bitter taste stimulates flow of saliva and digestive juices, increasing appetite

C

Carminative Relieves digestive gas, bloating, and indigestion

Circulatory stimulant Stimulates blood flow, usually to a given area, e.g. hands and feet

CITES Convention on International Trade and Endangered Species

Compress A cloth pad soaked in hot or cold herbal extract and applied firmly to the skin

Counterirritant Irritant to the skin used to relieve more deep-seated pain or discomfort

Cream A mixture of water with fat or oil that blends with the skin

D

Decoction Water-based preparation of root, bark, berries, or seeds simmered in boiling water

Demulcent Coats, soothes, and protects body surfaces such as the mucous membranes of the digestive tract

Depurative Detoxifying agent

Detoxification The process of aiding removal of toxins and waste products from the body, especially via liver and kidneys

Diaphoretic Induces sweating

Diuretic Stimulates urine flow

E

Emetic Causes vomiting

Emollient Softens or soothes the skin

Essential oil Aromatic oil distilled from plants containing volatile oils

Estrogenic Has estrogen-type hormonal activity within the body

Expectorant Stimulates more effective coughing and clearance of phlegm from the throat and chest

F

Fixed oil A nonvolatile oil (plant constituent). An oil produced by hot or cold infusion (preparation)

I

Immune modulator Promotes coordinated response by the body's immune defenses to counter infection and inflammation

Immune stimulant Stimulates the body's immune defenses to counter infection

Immunosuppressant Inhibits or blocks the body's normal immune defenses

Infusion Water-based preparation in which flowers, leaves, or stems are brewed in a similar way to tea

Inhalation Breathing of medicinally infused steam or liquid through the nasal passages

Interactions Where an herb and drug are taken at the same time, changing the effect of the drug (or herb), or producing an adverse reaction

L

Latex Sticky white or yellow juice released when plant part is broken, e.g. Dandelion leaf (Taraxacum officinale)

Laxative Promotes evacuation of the bowels

N

Nervine Restores the nerves, relaxes the nervous system

Neuralgia Pain caused by nerve irritation or damage

Nutritive Provides nutritional input

O

Ointment A blend of fats or oils that form a protective layer over the skin

P

Phytochemistry The study of plant chemistry—plant compounds and their makeup

Placebo A substance with no medicinal effect, used as a control in testing new medicines

Poultice Herbal preparation applied locally to alleviate pain or swelling

S

Sedative Reduces activity and nervous excitement

Spasmolytic Relaxes muscles

Standardized extract Herbal extract produced with defined level of key constituent(s)

Stimulant Increases rate of activity and nervous excitement

Synergy Where the combined effect, e.g. of an herbal remedy, is greater than the sum of the effects of its constituents

Synthetic Chemicals or medicines produced artificially in a laboratory rather than derived from natural products

Systemic Affecting the whole body

T

Tincture Liquid herbal preparation made by soaking herb in water and alcohol

Tonic Exerts a restorative or stimulant action on the body

Topical Application of herbal remedy to body surface

Tranquilizer Has relaxing and sedative properties

Tuber A swollen part of an underground stem, e.g. potato

V

Volatile oil Plant constituent distilled to produce essential oil

W

Wild crafting Gathering herb material from wild rather than cultivated plants

Resources

FINDING AN HERBAL PRACTITIONER

Herbal advice and medicines from a caring and knowledgeable professional can be invaluable when you are looking for a natural approach to health problems. Finding a well-qualified and professionally registered medical herbalist is not always easy. Recommendations from family and friends are helpful but you should always check that your practitioner is professionally registered. Members of the following associations are governed by a strict code of ethics and have all received intensive training in herbal and medical sciences, although the exact requirements for practicing herbal medicine vary, even within the US.

American Herbalists Guild (AHG)
141 Nob Hill Road
Cheshire, CT 06410
www.americanherbalistsguild.com
Largest professional association of herbalists in the US. Useful links on website include a complete guide to herbal training courses in North America and an explanation of the various credentials offered by herbalists in the US and internationally.

American Herbal Products Association (AHPA)
8484 Georgia Avenue
Silver Spring, MD 20910
www.ahpa.org
The only national trade association in the US that serves and represents growers and producers of herbs and herbal products. Web site includes "FAQs" for the herb user.

National Institute of Medical Herbalists
Elm House
54 Mary Arches Street
Exeter FX4 3BA
www.nimh.org.uk
Largest and oldest professional association of medical herbalists in the UK, with members throughout the UK and worldwide. Useful links on website, including information on training courses.

College of Practitioners of Phytotherapy
Oak Glade
9 Hythe Close
Polegate
East Sussex BN26 6LQ.
www. phytotherapists.org
Publishes the *British Journal of Phytotherapy*. Key scientific links on website.

European Herbal Practitioners Association (EHPA)
8 Lion Yard
Tremadoc Road
London SW4 7NQ
www.ehpa.eu
An "umbrella" organization for practitioner associations within the European Union.

IRELAND
Irish Institute of Medical Herbalists
www.iimh.org
Irish Medical Herbalists Organisation
http://www.mkdesign.ie/imho.html
Both organizations provide lists of well-qualified herbal practitioners.

AUSTRALIA
National Herbalists Association of Australia (NHAA)
4 Cavendish Street
Concord West NSW 2138
www.nhaa.org.au
Australia's oldest natural therapies association and only national professional body of medical herbalists. Website offers information on training courses and seminars, provides an herbal medicines discussion board, and allows you to search for an herbalist in your area.

NEW ZEALAND
New Zealand Association of Medical Herbalists (NZAMH)
PO Box 12582
Hamilton
www.nzamh.org.nz
New Zealand's organization of professional medical herbalists. Read the latest articles about herbal medicines or find a herbalist in your area.

HERBAL MEDICINE SUPPLIERS
US
There are many suppliers; to determine whether it is a reliable source, you should be able to confirm the following three points, whether you are in a store or purchasing herbal supplies online.
Does the company have certificates of analysis? Is a lot number and expiration date printed on every bottle? Does a complete list of all ingredients appear on every bottle?

Allergy Research Gropu
www.nutricology.com

Anabolic Laboratories
www.anaboliclabs.com

BioNativus
www.bionativus.com

Davinci Laboratories
www.davincilabs.com

Ethical Nutrients
www.ethicalnutrients.com

Gaia Herbs
www.gaiaherbs.com

Nature's Herbs
wwwnaturesherbs.com

UK
G. Baldwin & Co.
171/173 Walworth Road
London SE17 1RW
www.baldwins.co.uk
Wide range of herbs and tinctures, also mail order.

AUSTRALIA
Austral Herbs
Noalimba Ave
Kentucky NSW 2354
www.australherbs.com.au
Comprehensive online shop, supplying dried herbs, spices, and botanicals to customers worldwide.

NEW ZEALAND
New Zealand Herbals
26 Conway Street
Christchurch 8002

www.nzherbal.com
Provides natural healthcare services and products, with an extensive range of herbal supplements. Purchase herbal remedies, creams, and ointments online.

HERBAL INTEREST
The Herb Society
Sulgrave Manor
Sulgrave
Banbury OX17 2SD
www.herbsociety.org.uk
The Herb Society aims to promote interest in all aspects of herbal medicine—medicinal, culinary, and horticultural. It runs a national herb garden in Sulgrave, Northamptonshire, plus local groups, meetings, and conferences. Website has useful information, discussion board, and good links. It also lists other herb societies worldwide. A key organization for everyone interested in herbal medicine, it also publishes *Herbs*.

TRAINING COURSES
Discovering Herbal Medicine
www.newvitality.org.uk
A one-year correspondence course suitable for anyone interested in learning more about herbs and how to use them safely and confidently in their daily life. The course has been running for over 25 years and has been regularly updated. Highly recommended.

OTHER WEBSITES AND CONTACTS
American Botanical Council
www.herbalgram.org
A key international resource, with lots of useful information and links.
Publishes *Herbalgram*, perhaps the most informative English-language publication for those interested in herbal medicine.

Chelsea Physic Garden
66 Royal Hospital Road
London SW3 4HS
www.chelseaphysicgarden.co.uk
London's oldest medicinal herb garden in the middle of Chelsea.

Medline
www.nlm.nih.gov
Essential database for accessing scientific papers on herbal medicine.

Index

A

aches and pains 262, 266, 268, 275
  bogbean 166
  cramp bark 242
  lavender 152
  meadowsweet 160
  willow bark 196
  wild yam 116
acid indigestion 16, 262
  German chamomile 98
  meadowsweet 130
  slippery elm 232
Achillea millefolium 54
acne and boils 267
  burdock 72
  calendula 86
  echinacea 119
  tea tree 163
Actaea racemosa 100
adaptogen 125
  astragalus 73
  codonopsis 96
  ginseng 176
  schisandra 201
  Siberian ginseng 124
  withania 249
adrenal tonic
  licorice 141
adverse reactions 42, 43
Aesculus hippocastanum
  56–57, 58–59
alfalfa 162
allergic rhinitis *see* hay fever
allergy/allergies/allergic
  reactions 42, 259, 274
  baical skullcap 204
  blackcurrant 187
  eyebright 129
  German chamomile 98
Allium sativum 60–61
Aloe vera 36, 62–63, 64–65
Aloysia triphylla 157
alpha-linoleic acid 158, 159
Althea officinalis 66
anemia 264
  codonopsis 96
  nettle 235
Andrographis paniculata 55
Angelica archangelica 67
Angelica sinensis 68
anorexia nervosa 241
anxiety 271
  betony 210

lavender 152
lemon balm 164
limeflower 224
passion flower 173
sage 200
St. John's wort 148
skullcap 205
valerian 240
vervain 241
Apium graveolens 69
appetite, poor 262, 275
  bogbean 166
  dandelion 215
  gentian 136
Arctic root 186
Arctium lappa 70–71, 72
arnica 36, 66
Arnica montana 66
Artemisia annua 22
arthritic problems
  black cohosh 101
  bogbean 166
  boswellia 82
  celery 69
  devil's claw 145
  feverfew 213
  licorice 140
  nettle 234
  prickly ash 250
  turmeric 112
ashwagandha 249
Asian red sage 197
astragalus 73
Astragalus membranaceus
  73
atherosclerosis
  globe artichoke 113
  hawthorn 111
  limeflower 225
  sea buckthorn 146
Avena sativa 74
Azadirachta indica 75

B

back problems 266
  bacopa 76
Bacopa monniera 76
bacterial infection
  echinacea 118
  pau d'arco 214
  wild indigo root 76
bahupatra 180
baical skullcap 204
Baptisia tinctoria 76
barley 37
Barosma betulina 80
basil 167

benign prostatic hypertrophy
  (BPH)
  nettle root 234
  pumpkin seed 109
  saw palmetto 206
Berberis aquifolium 77
betony 210
Betula alba 81
bilberry 237
birch 81
black catnip 180
black cohosh 100–101
blackcurrant 187
bladder 265
bladderwrack 134
bleeding 191, 268, 269
bleeding, heavy menstrual
  raspberry 191
  yarrow 54
blood cleanser
  burdock 72
  dandelion 215
  nettle 234
  yellow dock 194
blood, common problems
  264–265
blood sugar levels 19, 264
  fenugreek 230
  holy basil 167
blueberry 237
body building
  puncture vine 223
bogbean 166
boils 267
bone, common problems 266
borage 78–79, 80
Borago officinalis 78–79, 80
boswellia 82
Boswellia serrata 82
breast-feeding
  and contraindications 43
  herbs commonly used 46
  herbs to avoid 46
breasts, sore 269
breath, shortness of 261
bronchial infection *see* chest
  infection
bruises 266, 267
  arnica 66
  comfrey 211
  witch hazel 144
buchu 86
bupleurum 83
Bupleurum falcatum 83
burdock 70–71, 72
burns 36, 268
  aloe vera 62

lavender 153
butcher's broom 192–193, 194
butterbur 178

C
cabbage 37
cacoa 218
caffeine 105, 172
calendula 84–85, 86
Calendula officinalis 84–85, 86
Californian poppy 126–127, 128
caltrops 223
Camellia sinensis 88–89
cancer
  black cohosh 101
  garlic 61
  pomegranate 180
  sheep's sorrel 194
  Siberian ginseng 125
  turmeric 112
  withania 249
cancer, anti-
  cat's claw 233
  golden root 186
  reishi 135
  shiitake 151
anti-inflammatory
  cat's claw 233
  ginger 255
  turmeric 112
  willow bark 196
capillary fragility
  bilberry 237
  witch hazel 144
Capsicum spp. 90–91, 92–93
capsules 28, 32, 45
caraway 94
cardamom 122
cardiovascular problems *see* circulatory porblems
Carduus marianus 207
Carica papaya 94
Curum carvi 94
Cassia spp. 87
catarrh 259, 261, 274
  eyebright 129
  fennel 131
  goldenseal 147
  limeflower 224
  plantain 181
  sage 200
cat's claw 233
cautions 16, 42, 43, 45, 260–275

cayenne pepper 37, 90–91, 92–93
celery 69
Centella asiatica 95
chai hu 83
Chamaelirium luteum 96
chamomile 98–99
Chamomilla recutita 98–99
chaste berry 244–245
chest infections
  butterbur 178
  cat's claw 233
  elecampane 150
  garlic 60
  licorice 140
  thyme 222
chest problems 261, 273–274
  cardamom 122
  coltsfoot 231
  heartsease 243
  lobelia 157
  red clover 226
chickweed 212
childbirth, aid
  raspberry 191
children
  common health problems 273–275
  suitable herbal remedies for 47
children's ailments
  Californian poppy 128
  German chamomile 99
chili 90–91, 92–93
Chinese angelica 68
Chinese wormwood 22
chocolate 218
cholesterol levels, raised 264
  fenugreek 230
  globe artichoke 113
  soy 137
chronic illness/infection 272
  blackcurrant 187
  cat's claw 233
  goldenseal 147
  Siberian ginseng 125
chronic inflammation 266
  boswellia 82
  licorice 140
  rehmannia 184
  turmeric 112
chronic skin disorders
  borage 80
  dandelion 215
  red clover 227
  yellow dock 195
chronic stress 271

chronic toxicity
  red clover 226
Cimicifuga racemosa 100–101
Cinnamomum verum 19, 97
cinnamon 19, 37, 97
circulation/circulatory
  problems 263–264
  blackcurrant 187
  bilberry 237
  chili 90
  dan shen 197
  garlic 61
  ginger 254
  ginkgo 138
  grape vine 248
  hawthorn 111
  horse chestnut 56–57
  limeflower 225
  mistletoe 243
  motherwort 156
  prickly ash 250
  rosemary 190
  yarrow 54
Citrus limon 102–103, 104
clinical trials 19
clove 37, 123
clover leaf 227
codonopsis 96
Codonopsis pilosula 96
Coffea arabica 105
coffee 30, 105
colds 261, 270, 274
  butterbur 178
  cinnamon 97
  chiretta 55
  echinacea 118
  elder 202
  ginger 255
  eucalyptus 128
  limeflower 224
  yarrow 54
coleus 106
Coleus forskohlii 106
Colic
  fennel 131
  German chamomile 99
  lemon balm 164
comfrey 36, 211
Commiphora molmol 36, 107
Commiphora mukul 107
concentration, poor 272
congestion 259, 261, 274
  elder 202
  elecampane 150
conjunctivitis 260, 273
constipation 262, 270, 275

linseed 158
rhubarb 185
senna 87
tamarind 214
yellow dock 194
contact allergy 45
contraindications 42–43
convalescence
alfalfa 162
elecampane 150
ginseng 176
Convallaria majalis 108
cordials 32
corn fronds 251
cornsilk 251, 252–253
coronary artery disease
hawthorn 110
coughs 261, 274
butterbur 178
caraway 94
coltsfoot 231
elecampane 150
eucalyptus 128
fennel 131
licorice 140
thyme 222
cramp bark 242
cramps 262, 268, 275
caraway 94
cramp bark 242
German chamomile 98
passion flower 173
peppermint 165
wild yam 116
cranberry 37, 236
Crataegus spp. 110–111
crataeva 108
Crataeva nurvala 108
creams 33, 36
Cucurbita pepo 109
Curcuma longa 112
cuts 36, 267
Cynara scolymus 113, 114–115
cystitis 265 *see also* urinary
tract problems

D

damiana 231
dan shen 197
dandelion 215, 216–217
dang shen 96
debility
alfalfa 162
decoctions 31, 44
preparing 34
dental treatment 260
depression

damiana 231
St. John's wort 148
depressed mood 271
golden root 186
detox remedies 268
burdock 72
celery 69
echinacea 119
lemon 104
turmeric 112
devil's claw 145
diarrhea 262, 275
digestion, poor/weak
bogbean 166
dandelion 215
gentian 136
hops 146
papaya 94
rosemary 190
digestive infection 262, 275
chili 91
clove 123
goldenseal 147
oregano 171
digestive problems 262, 263
angelica 66
bacopa 76
basil 167
calendula 86
chili 91
chiretta 55
cinnamon 97
cramp bark 242
German chamomile 98, 99
ginger 255
lavender 152
linseed 158
myrrh 107
Oregon grape 77
Digitalis purpurea 108
Dioscorea villosa 116–117
dizziness 259
black cohosh 100
ginkgo 138
dog rose 184
dong quai 68
dosage 42, 44–45, 258,
273
dried herbs 35, 50, 51
drug and herb interactions
43, 45
drying herbs 27

E

ear problems/infections 259
elder 202
goldenseal 147

lavender 152
tea tree 163
thyme 222
earache 259, 273
echinacea 36, 118–119,
120–121
Echinacea spp. 36, 118–119,
120–121
eczema 267
calendula 86
chickweed 212
gotu cola 95
heartsease 243
licorice
oats 74
sarsaparilla
elder 202–203
elecampane 150
Elettaria cardamomum 122
Eleutherococcus senticosus
124
emotional problems 271–272
emergency medical attention
42
endurance, physical
golden root 186
ginseng 176
Siberian ginseng 124
erectile dysfunction 270
Eschscholzia californica
126–127, 128
Essaic formula 194
essential oils 31, 33, 38, 45,
153
eucalyptus 128
Eucalyptus globulus 128
Eugenia caryophyllata 123
Euphrasia officinalis 129
evening primrose 168–169,
170
exams 17, 272
exhaustion
Siberian ginseng 124
withania 249
eye disorders/problems 260,
273
bilberry 237
eyebright 129
sea buckthorn 146
tea 88
witch hazel 144
eyebright 129
eyesight aid 260
bilberry 237

F

false unicorn root 96

fennel 131, 132–133
fenugreek 230
fertility, helping 269
fever 274
 elder 202
 limeflower 225
 willow bark 196
 yarrow 54
feverfew 213
fibromyalgia
 meadowsweet 130
 prickly ash 250
Filipendula ulmaria 130
first aid kit 36
fixed oils 33
flax 158–159
flax oil 159
flu 261, 270, 274
 chiretta 55
 echinacea 118
 elder 202
 yarrow 54
fluid retention
 dandelion leaf 215
Foeniculum vulgare 131,
 132–133
food supplements 23
fractures 266
freeze-dried extracts 33
frequency of urination 265
Fucus vesiculosis 134
fungal disorders/infection
 267
 lemon 104
 pau d'arco 214
 tea tree 163

G
gall-bladder, supporting 262
Ganoderma lucidum 135
garlic 36, 60–61
garlic oil 61
gas and bloating 262, 275
 cardamom 122
 fennel 131
 globe artichoke 113
 lemon balm 164
 peppermint 165
gastritis
 goldenseal 147
 licorice 140
 meadowsweet 130
 St. John's wort 149
gastrointestinal problems
  see digestive infection or
  problems
gelatine capsules 32

gentian 136
Gentiana luti 136
Gerard 245
German chamomile 98–99
ginger 30, 37, 254–255
ginkgo 138–139
Ginkgo biloba 138–139
ginseng 176–177
globe artichoke 113, 114 115
Glycine max 137
Glycyrrhiza glabra 140–141
golden root 186
goldenseal 147
gotu kola 95
grape vine 246–247, 248
grazes 36, 267
guarana 172
guelder rose 242
guggul 107
gum problems 260
gurmar 136
gymnema 136
Gymnema sylvestris 136
gynecological problems
 black cohosh 100
 helonias 96
 white peony 172

H
hair tonic
 nettle 235
 rosemary 190
Hamamelis virginiana 36,
 142–143, 144
Harpagophytum procumbens
 145
hawthorn 110–111
hay fever 259, 274
 butterbur 178
 elderflower 202
 eyebright 129
head, common problems
 259–260
 children 273–274
head lice 268
headache 259, 273
 betony 210
 coffee 105
 feverfew 213
 lavender 152
 lemon balm 164
 passion flower 173
 peppermint 165
 rosemary 190
 skullcap 205
healing, poor 264
health

and performance,
  promoting 272
 enhancing 17
 herbal 16–17
 problems that herbalists
  treat best 49
heart
 common problems
  263–264
 coleus 106
 dan shen 197
 lily of the valley 108
 hawthorn 110
 motherwort 156
heart, racing
 passion flower 173
heartsease 243
Helicobacter pylori 19, 97
helonias 96
hemorrhoids 264, 270
 witch hazel 144
herb garden 38–39
herbal dispensary 49
herbal medicine 14–15
 around the world 22–23
 making 26–27, 28–29
 types of 30–31, 32–33
herbal practitioners 19, 23,
 49, 50
herbal preparations, making
 simple 34–35
herbal remedies 14–15, 20–
 21, 23
 active constituents 21
 buying 50–51
 choosing the right 48
 combining 48
 for first aid kit 36
 home herbal 36, 37
 how long to take for 48
 making simple
  preparations 34–35
 safety of 16, 18–19, 42–43
 taking long term 17
 tips for home use 48–49
 when/how much to take 48
herbal tea, preparing 34
herb-drug interactions 43, 45
herbs 15
 growing 38–39
 harvesting and drying 27
 recommended plants to
  grow 38
 storing 21
herpes sores 267
high blood pressure
 cramp bark 242

dan shen 197
dandelion 215
hawthorn 110–111
limeflower 225
yarrow 54
Hippophae rhamnoides 146
hoarseness 16, 261
honey 37
hops 146
hormone therapy 227
hormones from wild yam 117
horse chestnut 56–57, 58–59
Humulus lupulus 146
Hydrastis canadensis 147
Hydrocotyle asiatica 95
Hypericum perforatum 28,
    43, 148–149

I

illness, preventing 17
immune support 272
    astralagus 73
    bupleurum 83
    blackcurrant 189
    chiretta 55
    echinacea 119
    withania 249
Indian frankincense 82
indigestion 262, 275
    fennel 131
    meadowsweet 130
infections 261, 262, 274
    echinacea 118
    garlic 60
    sea buckthorn 146
    thuja 219
infertility 270
    chaste berry 244
inflammation, chronic 266
inflammatory arthritis
    boswellia 82
    licorice 140
inflammatory bowel disease
    licorice 140
    turmeric 112
inflammatory conditions
    evening primrose 170
    German chamomile 98–99
infusions 31
injuries
    arnica 66
insect bites and stings 16
insomnia *see* sleep problems
interviews 17
Inula helenium 150
iodine 134
irritability

lavender 152
irritable bowel 262
    clove 123
    globe artichoke 113
    meadowsweet 130
    peppermint 165
    plantain 181
isoflavone extracts 227
itchy skin 267
    chickweed 212

J K

joints 266
    see also arthritic problems,
        rheumatic problems
juices 31
kelp 134
kidney problems
    birch 81
    bogbean 166
    crataeva 108
    globe artichoke 113
    grape vine 248
    puncture vine 223

L

lapacho 214
Lavandula spp. 36, 152–153,
    154–155
lavender 152–153, 154–155
lavender essential oil 36, 153
lemon 102–103, 104
lemon balm 164
lemon verbena 157
Lentinus edodes 151
Leonorus cardiaca 156
lily of the valley 108
limeflower 224–225
linctuses 32
linden blossom 224–225
ling-zhi 135
linseed 158–159, 160–161
linseed oil 159
Linum usitatissimum
    158–159, 160–161
Lippia citriodora 157
licorice 140–141
liver disorders 262
    black catnip 180
    chiretta 55
    dandelion 215
    globe artichoke 113
    goldenseal 147
    grape vine 248
    milk thistle 207
    schisandra 201
lobelia 157

Lobelia inflata 157
local pain relief
    lavender 152
local wound healing
    St. John's wort 149
low blood pressure
    hawthorn 110
    rosemary 190
low stamina
    Siberian ginseng 124
lucerne 162
lung conditions 261
    see also chest problems

M

mail order 50
malaria 22
male tonic
    cardamom 122
    ginseng 176
    puncture vine 223
    saw palmetto 206
marigold 86
marshmallow 66
Matricaria recutita 98
meadowsweet 130
Medicago sativa 162
medical herbalist 49
medicinal plants 14, 26–27
    active constituents 21
    and animals 20
    growing 38–39
    how they work 20
    research 19
Melaleuca alternifolia 163
melatonin 149
melissa 164
Melissa officinalis 164
memory, failing
    ginkgo 138
memory, poor 272
    sage 200
menopausal problems 269
    alfalfa 162
    black cohosh 100
    chaste berry 244
    fenugreek 230
    linseed 158
    parsley 179
    sage 200
    sarsaparilla 210
    soy 137
    red clover 227
    wild yam 116
men's health problems
    270–271
menstrual headache 259

menstrual bleeding 268, 269
  raspberry 191
menstrual disorders/
    problems
  chaste berry 244
  Chinese angelica 68
  cramp bark 242
  evening primrose 170
  German chamomile 98
  helonias 96
  motherwort 156
  skullcap 205
  white peony 172
  wild yam 116
mental problems 271–272
Mentha x piperita 165
metabolic, common
    problems 264–265
migraine 259, 273
  butterbur 178
  feverfew 213
  peppermint 165
  rosemary 190
milk thistle 207, 208–209
mistletoe 243
mood enhancement
  cacoa/chocolate 218
  damiana 231
  St. John's wort 148
monk's pepper 245
morning sickness 270
motherwort 156
motion sickness 262, 275
mouth ulcers 260, 274
  aloe vera 62
  licorice 140
  myrrh 107
  sage 200
mucilage 21
mucous membranes
    (soothing)
  marshmallow 66
  plantain 181
  slippery elm 232
muscular skeletal problems
    266
mushrooms see reishi,
    shiitake
mustard 90
myrrh 36, 107

N

National Institute of Medical
    Herbalists in the UK 49
natural progesterone cream
  wild yam 117
naturopaths 23

nausea 262, 275
  cinnamon 97
  German chamomile 98–99
  ginger 251
  peppermint 165
neem 75
nerve pain
  chili 90
  clove 123
  St. John's wort 149
nerve problems
  black cohosh 100
nervous debility/exhaustion
  betony 210
  damiana 231
  oats 74
  rosemary 190
  St. John's wort 148
  withania 249
nervous tension/disorders
    see also anxiety
  bacopa 76
  German chamomile 98
  limeflower 224
  mistletoe 243
  passion flower 173
  skullcap 205
  valerian 240
  vervain 241
nettle 234–235
nettle rash 267
nettle soup 235
nose infection 259
nose problems
  elder 202
  thyme 222
nosebleed 259, 274
nutritional supplements 18

O

oat straw 240
oats 74
Ocimum basilicum 167
Ocimum sanctum 167
Oenothera biennis 168–169,
    170
oils
  carrier 33
  essential 31, 33, 38, 45, 153
  fixed 33
  vegetable 33
  volatile 21
ointments 33, 36
olive oil 37
omega-3 essential fatty acids
    158, 159, 161
omega-6 fatty acids 80, 170,

    187
oregano 171
Oregon grape 77
oral thrush 260, 274
organic certification 27, 51
Origanum majorana 171
Origanum vulgare 171
osteoporosis 269
  black cohosh 100–101
  parsley 179
  withania 249

P

Paeonia lactiflora 172
pain relief
  butterbur 178
  Californian poppy 128
  lavender 152
  passion flower 173
  St. John's wort 149
pains see aches and pains
palpitations 263
  lemon balm 164
  limeflower 225
  motherwort 156
Panax ginseng 176–177
papain 94
papaya 94
parsley 179
passiflora 173, 174–175
Passiflora incarnata 173,
    174–175
passion flower 173, 174–175
pau d'arco 214
Paullinia cupana 172
paw paw 94
peppermint 165
peppers, chili 91
peptic ulcer
  licorice 140
performance, promoting 272
peripheral circulation 263
  bilberry 237
  dan shen 197
  ginger 254
  ginkgo 138
Petasites hybridus 178
Petroselinum crispum 179
Phyllanthus amarus 180
physical endurance
  golden root 186
  ginseng 176
phytoestrogens 137, 158
Plantago spp. 181
plantain 181
PMS see premenstrual
    syndrome

polycystic ovary syndrome 206
  chaste berry 244
  licorice 141
  saw palmetto 206
  white peony 172
powders 33, 45
pregnancy 46–47, 270
  and contra-indications 43
  herbs commonly used 46
  herbs to avoid 46
  raspberry 191
premenstrual syndrome
    (PMS)
  black cohosh 100
  chaste berry 244
  skullcap 205, 268
  vervain 241
preventing illness 17
prickly ash 250
professional advice 16, 49
prostate 271
  cranberry 236
  nettle 234
  saw palmetto 206
pumpkin seed 109
puncture vine 223
Punica granatum 180

R
racing heart
  passion flower 173
  raspberry 191
red clover 226–227, 228–229
reflux 262
rehmannia 184
Rehmannia glutinosa 184
reishi 135
respiratory disease see chest
    problems
respiratory infection see
    chest infections
restless legs 266
rheumatic aches and pains
    see aches and pains
rheumatic problems
  birch 81
  black cohosh 101
  bogbean 166
  devil's claw 145
  nettle 234
  prickly ash 250
Rheum officinalis 185
Rhodiola rosea 186
rhubarb 185
Ribes nigrum 187
Rosa spp. 182–183, 184
rose 182–183, 184

rosemary 188–189, 190
rosewater 182, 184
Rosmarinus officinalis
    188–189, 190
Rubus ideaus 191
Rumex acetosella 194
Rumex crispus 195
Ruscus aculeatus 192–193,
    194

S
SAD see seasonal affective
    disorder
safety of herbal remedies
    18–19, 42–43
  see also cautions
sage 198–199, 200
St. John's wort 28, 43,
    148–149
Salix alba 196
Salvia miltiorrhiza 197
Salvia lavandulifolia 200
Salvia officinalis 198–199,
    200
Sambucus nigra 202–203
sarsaparilla 210
saw palmetto 206
schisandra 201
Schisandra chinesis 201
sciatica
  St. John's wort 149
scientific research 19, 20
Scutellaria baicalensis 204
Scutellaria lateriflora 205
sea buckthorn 146
seasonal affective disorder
    (SAD) 271
  St. John's wort 148
self-treatment 15, 48
senna 87
Serenoa repens 206
sexual tonic
  damiana 231
  puncture vine 223
  saw palmetto 206
  sheep's sorrel 194
  shiitake 151
shingles 267
  St. John's wort 149
shortness of breath 261
Siberian ginseng 124–125
side effects 16, 19, 42
Silybum marianum 207,
    208–209
Sinapsis alba 90
sinuses 259
skin conditions/problems

    267–269
  aloe vera 62
  borage 80
  calendula 86
  dandelion 215
  evening primrose 170
  eucalyptus 128
  heartsease 243
  myrrh 107
  neem 75
  nettle 234
  Oregon grape 77
  sarsaparilla 210
  tea tree 163
skin toner
  rosewater 184
  witch hazel 144
skullcap 205
sleep difficulties 271
  Californian poppy 128
  lavender 152
  lemon verbena 157
  limeflower 224
  hops 146
  passion flower 173
  St. John's wort 148
  valerian 240
slippery elm 36, 232
Smilax spp. 210
snake root 119
sore breasts 269
sore eyes/lids 260, 273
sore throat 16, 261, 274
  fennel 131
  licorice 140
  sage 200
soy 137
Spanish sage 200
sports injuries 266
sprains 266
  comfrey 211
squaw root 101
Stachys officinalis 210
standardized extracts 28
starflower 80
Stellaria media 212
stevia 212
Stevia rebaudiana 212
stomach ache 275
stomach ulcer
  St. John's wort 149
stress 271
  sage 200
  see also anxiety, and
    nervous exhaustion
stress, long-term
  ginseng 176

golden root 186
Siberian ginseng 124
styes 260, 273
sugar craving
gymnema 136
sugar replacement 212
sugar tolerance, poor
gymnema 136
sunburn 268
Symphytum officinale 211
symptoms 42
and choice of remedy 48
and professional help 49
syrups 32
Syzygium aromaticum 123

T U

Tabebuia spp. 214
tablets 23, 32–33, 45
tamarind 214
Tamarindus indica 214
Tanacetum parthenium 213
Taraxacum officinalis 216–217
tea 88–89
tea drinking 89
tea tree 36, 163
tea, herbal 31, 45
tension headache 259, 273
betony 210
lavender 152, 153
lemon balm 164
limeflower 224
Theobroma cacao 218
thread veins
witch hazel 144
throat problems 261
aloe vera 62
cardamom 122
elder 202
thyme 222
fennel 131
licorice 140
sage 200
thrush 269
mouth 260, 274
thuja 219
Thuja occidentalis 219
thyme 36, 220–221, 222
Thymus vulgaris 220–221, 222
thyroid gland
overactive 265
underactive 265
bladderwrack/kelp 134
Tilia spp. 224–225
tincture 32, 45, 50

preparing 34
tinnitus 259
black cohosh 100
ginkgo 138
tissue, broken or inflamed
aloe vera 62
gotu kola 95
plantain 181
yarrow 54
tissue repair
comfrey 211
toothache 260, 273
clove 123
St. John's wort 149
tree of life 219
Tribulus terrestris 223
Trifolium pratense 226–227, 228–229
Trigonella foenum-graecum 230
tulsi 167
turmeric 112
Turnera aphrodisiaca 231
Turnera diffusa 231
Tussilago farfara 231
Ulmus fulva 232
una de gato 233
Uncaria tomentosa 233
urinary tract problems 265
buchu 80
cornsilk 251
cranberry 236
marshmallow 66
parsley 179
puncture vine 223
saw palmetto 206
Urtica dioica 234–235
Urtica urens 234

V

Vaccinium macrocarpon 236
Vaccinium myrtillis 237
vaginal infection
tea tree 163
valerian 238, 239, 240
Valeriana officinalis 238–239, 240
varicose veins 264, 270
butcher's broom 194
horse chestnut 56
witch hazel 144
varuna 108
vegetable oil 33
veins/venous insufficiency
butcher's broom 194
horse chestnut 56, 57
Veratrum luteum 96

Verbena officinalis 241
vervain 241
Viburnum opulus 242
vinegar 32
Viola tricolor 243
viral infection
black catnip 180
echinacea 118
elderflower/berry 202
ginger 255
licorice 140
thuja 219
Viscum album 243
vitamin C 187, 202
Vitex agnus-castus 244–245
Vitis vinifera 246–247, 248
volatile oils 21
vomiting
ginger 251

W Y Z

warts 267
thuja 219
weight gain 262
weight loss 262
white peony 172
white willow 196
wild-crafting 26–27
wild indigo root 76
wild marjoram 171
wild pansy 243
wild plants, picking of 26
wild yam 116–117
willow bark 196
winter blues 271
St. John's wort 148
witch hazel 36, 142–143, 144
withania 249
Withania somniferum 249
women's health 268–269
worms 262, 275
wounds 267
aloe vera 62
comfrey 211
gotu kola 95
St. John's wort 149
wu wei zi 201
yarrow 54
yellow dock 195
Zanthoxylum clava-herculis 250
Zea mays 251, 252–253
Zingiber officinalis 30, 254–255